STUDY GUIDE TO ACCOMPANY

BREASTFEEDING AND HUMAN LACTATION   THIRD EDITION

Mary-Margaret Coates, MS, IBCLC
Galactaguide
Wheat Ridge, Colorado

Jan Riordan, EdD, RN, IBCLC, FAAN
School of Nursing
Wichita State University
Wichita, Kansas

JONES AND BARTLETT PUBLISHERS
Sudbury, Massachusetts
BOSTON   TORONTO   LONDON   SINGAPORE

World Headquarters
Jones and Bartlett Publishers
40 Tall Pine Drive
Sudbury, MA 01776
978-443-5000
info@jbpub.com
www.jbpub.com

Jones and Bartlett Publishers Canada
6339 Ormindale Way
Mississauga, ON L5V 1J2
CANADA

Jones and Bartlett Publishers International
Barb House, Barb Mews
London W6 7PA
UK

Copyright © 2005 by Jones and Bartlett Publishers, Inc.

Cover image © InJoy Productions, Inc.
Section 2 opener © Humenick, 1987.
Section 5 opener © Kathleen G. Auerbach.

ISBN-13: 978-0-7637-2703-1
ISBN-10: 0-7637-2703-2

Acquisitions Editor: Kevin Sullivan
Production Manager: Amy Rose
Associate Production Editor: Jenny L. McIsaac
Editorial Assistant: Amy Sibley
Marketing Manager: Edward McKenna
Associate Marketing Manager: Emily Ekle
Manufacturing Buyer: Amy Bacus
Cover Design: Colleen Halloran
Composition: Interactive Composition Corporation
Printing and Binding: Malloy, Inc.
Cover Printing: Malloy, Inc.

Printed in the United States of America
11 10 09 08 07   10 9 8 7 6 5 4 3 2

This book is dedicated to the memory of my mother, Martha Seem Hepp, who paid attention when her family doctor, Fred C. Rewerts, MD, said, "Aw, Martha, breastfeed 'em; they just do better," and went on to breastfeed three children in the late 1930s and early 1940s.

Mary-Margaret Coates

TABLE OF CONTENTS

SUGGESTIONS FOR USING THIS STUDY GUIDE

This study guide, which accompanies the textbook *Breastfeeding and Human Lactation, Third Edition,* will help you assess your current knowledge of human lactation and prepare you for certification as a lactation consultant.

The study guide is organized to correspond with the third edition of the text *Breastfeeding and Human Lactation* by Jan Riordan, published in 2004 by Jones and Bartlett Publishers. Every question (and its answer) in this study guide is tied to information in the third edition. Each chapter in this study guide contains the following:

- An outline of the corresponding chapter in the textbook.

- Multiple-choice questions that test the reader's understanding of facts about lactation and breastfeeding. Answers are in the back of the book.

- Discussion questions that may or may not have a single best answer but are designed to spark discussion and prompt review of the topic addressed.

As compared with the previous edition of the study guide, this edition contains many more multiple-choice questions and fewer discussion questions. This realignment of question types will better prepare you both for the IBLCE examination and for problems that you will encounter in clinical practice. Also, more questions are posed on topics emphasized in the IBLCE exam. Either type of question can be used to generate discussions in exam study groups, "brown-bag" staff meetings, and journal clubs.

About the Questions in This Study Guide

Multiple-Choice Questions

Multiple-choice questions can sometimes be tedious to work through or tricky to interpret. Here are some tips to smooth the way:

- Each question begins with a stem—either a question or the beginning of a statement—followed by four options that either answer the question or complete the statement.

- Each question has *one best* answer mixed in with the other options.

- In many cases, you will be able to quickly eliminate one or two obviously incorrect answers. Now you must ferret out the *one best* response from the remaining, partially correct alternatives.

    If you consistently pick correct answers, congratulations! If you don't, try to figure out what went wrong. Did you misread the question? Did you read only part of the possible answers, thereby selecting an alternative that was partially correct but not the one best answer? (Or maybe you just didn't know the right response.) If you answered incorrectly, go back and reread the question and the correct answer. If you don't understand why a given answer is considered correct (or if you disagree with that answer), review the topic in the chapter of the same name in *Breastfeeding and Human Lactation, Third Edition*.

Discussion Questions

The discussion questions require you to organize what you understand about a topic into a coherent form, so that you can explain the topic—to yourself, if you are working alone, or to your colleagues. No answers are provided to these questions because your answers can rightfully be influenced by your own experiences as a lactation consultant as well as by the textbook information.

Preparing for and Taking a Certification Exam

A certification examination will test two types of knowledge: what you know cognitively and how well you use that information when confronted with a problem. You will do best if you begin the test relaxed and ready to go–a state easier to achieve if you are well prepared.

The International Board of Lactation Consultant Examiners Examination

Most certification examinations, including the one administered by the International Board of Lactation Consultant Examiners, Inc. (IBLCE), consist of a long series of multiple-choice questions. Past IBLCE exams have contained about 200 questions. The certification examination is divided into morning and afternoon segments.

The morning session is devoted exclusively to multiple-choice questions. The test booklet contains all the information you need in order to answer each question; you can make notes in the booklet at will. You will record your answers on a separate machine-scorable answer sheet. On this answer sheet, be careful to mark the correct slot for the correct question. Because your total score is based on the number of correct answers (not the number of wrong answers), make educated guesses even if you don't know the correct answer.

You will have about 3 hours in which to complete the morning session. You may leave the examination room when you are finished. If you finish early, review questions about which you were unsure. Even if you are a slow test taker, you should have sufficient time to complete the morning segment. But if you run out of time before you run out of questions, you will lose points. If you tend to take tests slowly, practice answering multiple-choice questions with four possible answers within a set time–about one question per minute–so that you can get a feel for how quickly you should proceed through the real examination.

During the afternoon session you will answer multiple-choice questions keyed to illustrations in a second test booklet. Practice for this portion beforehand by looking at slides or photographs of breastfeeding situations and then answering questions about them–questions that you make up or questions provided by the vendor of the illustrations.

Because the IBLCE seeks to determine minimum competency, you need not have the top score in order to be certified. Usually the lowest passing score is in the middle to low 60th percentile.

Before an Exam

Give yourself plenty of time to study–weeks or months rather than three all-nighters right before the exam. If you think of the exam as a performance, you can appreciate that regular, frequent rehearsals are the best preparation.

Many successful certification candidates meet with colleagues once or twice a week for several months; commonly, each assumes responsibility for leading a discussion about a particular topic. Then they go through the study guide questions bearing on that chapter (or topic). Discussion questions can be used as a basis for writing additional multiple-choice questions.

The day before the exam, exercise vigorously enough so that you can relax and get a good night's sleep. Go to bed early; you will then be more alert and able to concentrate better on test day. On test-day morning, do yourself a favor: *Eat breakfast*! Taking a certification exam requires a lot of energy; you don't want to fade out mid-morning. Your breakfast should contain enough protein and calories to keep you going for several hours and should sit lightly in your stomach. This isn't the time to try out a new recipe or to include an ingredient that upset your stomach last week.

Staying Comfortable During an Exam

Sites: Examination sites differ. You may be asked to report to a hotel room, a college or hospital classroom, a church hall, or some other public meeting room not designed for test takers. Distracting noises may intrude into the room. Uneven lighting may make the exam hard to read or the illustrations difficult to see clearly. If such distractions are present, insist that your exam administrator make appropriate adjustments.

Clothing: Regardless of the season, it's best to dress in layers. Wear garments that you can easily put on or take off. Bring a sweater—meeting rooms are generally chilly. Dress for comfort instead of style. Wear loose, casual clothing that you would choose for a day-long plane ride or car trip.

Snacks and medicines: Physical discomfort, such as hunger, will distract you from the examination. If you are allowed to bring hard candies or other small snacks with you, do so. When you're struggling to think through a particularly knotty question, a bit of quick energy will help your performance. On the day of the exam, try to avoid taking medicines that make you drowsy.

Anxiety: If you feel panicky during the exam, try one or more of these techniques:

- Take several deep breaths. If you know breathing techniques for labor and childbirth, use them.
- Close your eyes and try to visualize yourself in a safe and relaxing place.
- Practice progressive relaxation by relaxing successive muscle groups. Begin with the tips of your toes and work up your body, or start at the top of your head and work down.
- If you feel your heart beating rapidly, tell yourself, "I'm going to breathe deeply, and my heart rate will slow." Then imagine your heart slowing as you breathe deeply and slowly several times.
- Some test takers say to themselves, "This is an easy exam" or "I know almost all of the answers" or "I know how to take this kind of exam." Such thoughts create a positive mindset.

No one has died from taking a certification exam. Enter the examination room alert to your surroundings and ready to concentrate on the task at hand. It's okay to feel a bit anxious—that feeling often will help give you a good "edge." Think of the exam questions as hurdles of differing heights, most of which you will easily sail over. Each time you answer a question, you've cleared a hurdle and you will gain confidence in your ability to continue successfully.

Test-Taking Strategies

General strategies: The following strategies may help you move through an exam with confidence:

- Approach each question as if it were your only care in the world. Read it carefully all the way to the end.
- Concentrate on the question at hand. Don't read information into the question or allow your mind to wander back to previous questions.
- Eliminate clearly incorrect options before selecting from the remaining alternatives.
- Skip questions that stump you; come back to them at the end. By that time your mind is warmed up and the answer often will come easily.
- Trust your intuition; trust yourself. Your first hunch is usually right.
- Use the test booklet to jot down notes.
- Select the one option that you think is the *best* response.
- Record your answer correctly on the answer sheet.
- Once you've completed a question, put it out of your mind.

Analyzing questions: Some general comments about analyzing multiple-choice questions are discussed above. Now, let's talk about the IBLCE exam in particular.

- Words like *always* and *never* will rarely be part of a correct answer.

- Look for questions that ask for *first* (or *last*) actions—for example, "What would you do first?" Although all of the choices offered may describe correct actions, the *one best* answer will be the response that you will make first (or last).

- Look at the question stem first. The stem tells you what you need to look for (in the following description or in an illustration) in order to pick the correct answer.

- Decide whether the stem is positive or negative before proceeding with the question. Note negative words and prefixes—for example, "All of the following are true EXCEPT" or "Not breastfeeding is associated with . . . ."

- Pace yourself. Try to complete each question within 1 minute. It is to your advantage to guess at remaining questions if you do not have time to analyze each of them.

- For a question coupled with an illustration, first read the stem of the question. The stem will direct your attention to particular aspects of the illustration. Now look briefly at the illustration and get a sense of what you are looking at (or for). Then sort through the possible answers, always looking for that *one best* answer.

Here are three examples of how to apply the techniques just described:

1. The most effective technique for using a textbook to study for an exam is to
   a. read the textbook as close to the exam date as possible.
   b. read the textbook a little at a time.
   c. write one or two questions that you think might be asked.
   d. concentrate on the summary information and the tables, if any.

   - Alternative a is clearly incorrect. Following its advice is likely to increase your anxiety and prevent you from getting through the material before the exam.
   - Alternative b is excellent advice, particularly when you are attempting to learn and remember a large body of information. It looks like it might be the *one best* answer—but don't stop here. Read all of the alternatives before you decide.
   - Alternative c is also good advice, but one or two questions are unlikely to be enough to help you remember what you've read. This answer is partially correct, but not the *one best* answer.
   - Alternative d is good advice, but summary information and tables are unlikely to include some of the more detailed information that you may need to know. It is partially correct, but not the *one best* answer.

2. When confronted by a multiple-choice question you don't understand,
   a. select the most difficult-to-understand alternative.
   b. go back to the question later.
   c. select the one option you do understand.
   d. guess at the answer.

   - Alternative a is a poor choice. The less you understand, the less likely you are to select the correct answer.

- Alternative b is a better choice. Time, relaxing a bit more, and getting into a test-taking mode may be all you need to understand the question more completely.

- Alternative c may be the best choice. The option you understand is more likely than others to be the correct answer. Remember, the test writers are not trying to trick you. But don't stop here—read all of the alternatives before you decide on your answer.

- Alternative d is a poor choice in practice if any other means are available. Improve your odds before guessing by eliminating any clearly incorrect alternatives. If you've reduced your choices to two then you have a 50–50 chance of guessing correctly. However, guessing from four options gives you only a 25 percent chance of correctly answering the question.

3. When you are taking a multiple-choice test that includes visual material, how should you approach the question?

   a. Look at the picture for at least 30 seconds and then read the question.

   b. Read the stem of the question first, look at the photo, and then read the options.

   c. Read the stem of the question and all of the options; then look at the photo.

   d. Look at the picture and then read the options.

   - Alternative a is a poor choice. Simply looking at the picture for a long period may not tell you what is being asked. You may lose valuable time following this advice.

   - Alternative b is a good choice. By reading the stem of the question, you may be given a clue about what to look for in the visual material. This will help you correctly select the right option. But don't stop here—read all of the alternatives before deciding on your answer.

   - Alternative c is a poor choice. If you spend too much time on the written portion of the question, you may not have enough time to examine the visual material.

   - Alternative d is also a poor choice. The visual material may, in the absence of awareness of the stem, give you an incorrect impression when selecting the options.

The Exam Is Over!

When you've completed the examination, celebrate having survived—and then try to forget about it. It will be many weeks before you learn how well you did. Until the day you receive your certificate declaring that you are now a certified lactation consultant, concentrate on the rest of your busy and fulfilling life.

Accompanying CD-ROM

At the back of this study guide you will find a CD-ROM which can also help you to prepare for certification exams. The CD includes the same multiple-choice questions that are printed in this study guide. Additional functionality allows you to sort the questions by chapter or randomize the questions. The correct answers to the questions are provided once you have entered your answers. Your overall score on the questions you have chosen to answer is also compiled. Please review the CD for further instructions.

Photo Library

The third edition of Breastfeeding and Human Lactation contains an electronic photo library which offers a number of photographs from the book on a CD-ROM. This photo library can help you prepare for the photo portion of the IBCLE exam.

ACKNOWLEDGMENTS

I wish to recognize the efforts and astute comments of the following reviewers of this study guide: Susannah Coates, Anna Marie Heard, Laraine Lockhart Borman, Mary Tagge, Darcy Kamin, and Kathy Kennedy. In addition, many thanks are due to Kathleen Auerbach, who prepared the study guide accompanying the second edition of this text.

Mary-Margaret Coates

AUTHORS OF CHAPTERS IN BREASTFEEDING AND HUMAN LACTATION, THIRD EDITION

1. Tides in Breastfeeding Practice

   Mary-Margaret Coates, MS, IBCLC
   Jan Riordan, EdD, RN, IBCLC, FAAN

2. Work Strategies and the Lactation Consultant

   Jan Riordan, EdD, RN, IBCLC, FAAN

3. Anatomy and Physiology of Lactation

   Jan Riordan, EdD, RN, IBCLC, FAAN

4. The Biological Specificity of Breastmilk

   Jan Riordan, EdD, RN, IBCLC, FAAN

5. Drug Therapy and Breastfeeding

   Thomas W. Hale, PhD, RPH

6. Viruses and Breastfeeding

   Jan Riordan, EdD, RN, IBCLC, FAAN

7. Perinatal and Intrapartum Care

   Jan Riordan, EdD, RN, IBCLC, FAAN
   Kay Hoover, MEd, IBCLC

8. Postpartum Care

   Linda J. Smith, BSE, FACCE, IBCLC
   Jan Riordan, EdD, RN, IBCLC, FAAN

9. Breast-Related Problems

   Jan Riordan, EdD, RN, IBCLC, FAAN

10. Low Intake in the Breastfed Infant: Maternal and Infant Considerations

    Nancy G. Powers, MD

11. Jaundice and the Breastfed Baby

    Marguerite Herschel, MD
    Lawrence M. Gartner, MD

12. Breast Pumps and Other Technologies

    Marsha Walker, RN, IBCLC

13. Breastfeeding the Preterm Infant

    Nancy M. Hurst, RN, MSN, IBCLC
    Paula P. Meier, DNSc, RN, FAAN

14. Donor Human Milk Banking

    Lois D.W. Arnold, PhD (C.), MPH, IBCLC

15. Maternal Nutrition During Lactation

    Yvonne L. Bronner, ScD, RD, LD
    Kathleen G. Auerbach, PhD, IBCLC

16. Women's Health and Breastfeeding

    Jan Riordan, EdD, RN, IBCLC, FAAN

17. Maternal Employment and Breastfeeding

    Karen A. Wambach, PhD, RN, IBCLC
    Wailaiporn Rojjanasrirat, PhD, MSN

18. Child Health

    Jan Riordan, EdD, RN, IBCLC, FAAN

HISTORICAL AND WORK PERSPECTIVES

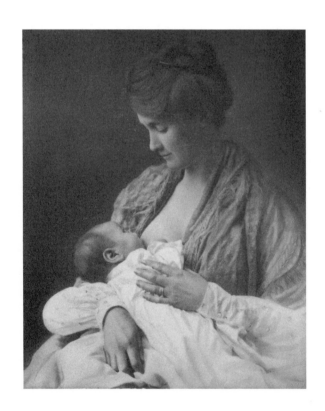

Tides in Breastfeeding Practice

This chapter tries to bridge some 70 million years of human history. On both an individual level (breastfeeding guidance) and a societal level (breastfeeding promotion) we aspire to achieve what was the norm many generations ago. Questions in this chapter will help you to put into a longer perspective the historical basis for modern breastfeeding practices and the goals we hope to achieve.

Chapter Outline

The Cost of Not Breastfeeding

    Health risks of using manufactured infant milks

    Economic costs of using manufactured infant milks

The Promotion of Breastfeeding

    Breastfeeding promotion in the United States

    International breastfeeding promotion

    Private support movements

Summary

Key Concepts

Internet Resources

References

Multiple-Choice Questions

1. Which of the following breastfeeding patterns is thought to have typified human groups before 10,000 B.C.?

    a. frequent but brief breastfeeding bouts, day and night

    b. total duration of breastfeeding of only a few months

    c. infrequent daytime breastfeeding bouts coupled with frequent nighttime bouts

    d. infrequent but long breastfeeding bouts

2. Humans belong to a class of animals (Mammalia) whose distinguishing characteristic is

    a. upright posture.

    b. breasts.

    c. forward-facing paired eyes.

    d. opposable thumbs.

3. Evidence shows that animal milks were used as an infant food

    a. very early–several million years ago–in the evolutionary history of *Homo sapiens.*

    b. first in industrialized countries shortly after the development of tinned milks.

    c. relatively recently–a few thousand years ago–after the development of animal husbandry.

    d. only when wet-nursing fell out of favor as an alternative to maternal nursing.

4. After weaning from the breast, an individual's ability to tolerate lactose

    a. is the worldwide norm.

    b. generally increases in societies that use animal milks as a food staple.

    c. generally remains high in societies that do not use animal milks as a food staple.

    d. generally diminishes in societies that do not use animal milks as a food staple.

5. Hand-feeding foods other than breastmilk before a neonate is put to breast is

    a. an uncommon practice except in highly industrialized societies.

    b. a common practice in both traditional and industrialized societies.

    c. an uncommon practice owing to concerns about the safety of such feeds.

    d. a common practice only in traditional societies.

6. Delay in putting a newborn to breast combined with early hand feeding is a set of practices that

    a. nearly always undermines breastfeeding in all societies.

    b. rarely undermines breastfeeding if it is encouraged by the mother's mother.

    c. rarely undermines breastfeeding in any society.

    d. rarely undermines breastfeeding if subsequent breastfeeding is supported by cultural expectation.

7. In the United States, the prevalence of breastfeeding

    a. has remained low since the early 1900s.

    b. declined in the late 1940s but has generally risen since the 1970s.

    c. has remained high since the early 1900s.

    d. has generally been high but is currently on the decline.

8. Worldwide and throughout history, the factor most strongly linked with infant mortality is

    a. a decline in rates of breastfeeding.

    b. poverty.

    c. use of Western-style feeding patterns in non-Western settings.

    d. the local advent of industrialization.

9. Declines in breastfeeding prevalence may not be mirrored by increases in infant mortality if

    a. infants are secluded in their families until they are 3 or 4 years old.

    b. the mother can read.

    c. widespread primary health care is available.

    d. the family diet contains enough calories.

10. As compared with the cost of bottle-feeding, the cost to a family of breastfeeding is

    a. lower, in part because the mother requires little extra food.

    b. higher, because the mother must consume high-quality foods in order to produce adequate milk.

    c. lower, because the breastfed infant on average consumes less milk than a bottle-fed infant.

    d. higher, because the mother must seek medical care more frequently.

11. As compared with infants fed manufactured milks, breastfed infants tend to have

    a. less illness because breastmilk immunoglobulins help the infant resist bacteria.

    b. less illness because the protein in breastmilk is more dilute.

    c. more illness because the nutritional status of artificially fed infants is better.

    d. more illness because of the relatively dilute nature of breastmilk.

12. The International Code of Marketing of Breast-Milk Substitutes
    a. forbids, while a mother and baby are in the hospital, the mother's use of manufactured milks.
    b. allows the public advertisement of manufactured milks.
    c. forbids government distribution directly to consumers of free manufactured milks.
    d. supports the right of hospitals to distribute free samples of manufactured milks.

13. The Baby-Friendly Hospital Initiative
    a. encourages mothers to obtain a full first-night's rest in the hospital.
    b. encourages hospitals to promote exclusive breastfeeding.
    c. is more easily implemented in industrialized nations because needed technology is available.
    d. requires less staff time to implement than does traditional nursery care of newborns.

Discussion Questions

1. What constitutes "normal" breastfeeding practices?

2. What is "wet-nursing"? Why is it rarely practiced in industrialized countries today?

3. What is "hand-feeding"? Name three hand-fed foods and describe their effect on the nutritional status and general health of a 1-month-old infant and on a 6-month-old infant.

4. What are prelacteal feeds? Offer at least three explanations for their use in various cultures or time periods.

5. How do you explain the relationship in many parts of the world between high breastfeeding rates and high infant mortality?

6. Identify and briefly discuss four different health risks resulting from the use of artificial baby milks. Explain why some health risks appear to be short term, whereas others are long term.

7. Briefly describe three levels of cost incurred by feeding manufactured milks to infants: the cost to a family, the cost to the family's community, and the broader cost to society. The word "cost" may be considered in financial or in other terms.

8. What is the WHO Code? Why is it important in a developing country? in a developed country?

9. Describe the steps in the Baby-Friendly Hospital Initiative.

10. Explain the role of advertising in increasing the use of manufactured baby milks. Give three examples of how these products are advertised to the public and to health-care professionals.

11. Identify how class differences in both an industrialized country and a nonindustrialized country have influenced the likelihood of breastfeeding initiation and its duration. If the patterns of behavior are different, how do you explain this difference?

12. What is breastfeeding promotion? Outline three ways in which breastfeeding might be promoted.

13. Explain why both the older and the younger infant are at greater risk for mortality when birth spacing is short.

14. Price the cost of 150 cans of ready-to-feed manufactured baby milk, about the number of cans used during a baby's first 6 months. What proportion of income must be assigned to the purchase of infant milk for a family whose monthly income is

    a. $500.   c. $2,500.

    b. $1,000.

15. Exclusive feeding of manufactured milk is likely to lead to what other expenditures? Estimate the cost of those other expenditures.

16. How would you implement each of the Ten Steps to Successful Breastfeeding in a health-care facility in your community? Which steps would you implement first? Why? How would you ensure that each step is implemented?

WORK STRATEGIES AND THE LACTATION CONSULTANT

Lactation consultants are specialists who extend maternal–child health care in many settings. Questions in this chapter will help you assess your familiarity with practical ways that a lactation consultant can meet her professional and legal responsibilities to the mother and baby she is assisting, to her employer, and to society at large.

Chapter Outline

Multiple-Choice Questions

1. Most research studies on the effect of lactation consultant advice to a breastfeeding mother show that
   a. casual advice does not increase the prevalence or duration of breastfeeding.
   b. lactation consultant advice can increase duration but not initiation of breastfeeding.
   c. almost any exchange between lactation consultants and new mothers increases the duration of breastfeeding.
   d. in rural populations, lactation consultant advice may or may not promote breastfeeding, whereas in metropolitan populations it does.

2. Long-established hospital routines used for the care of a breastfeeding dyad are
   a. easy to change when the changes are supported by substantial research.
   b. easy to change because most staff want to keep up to date.
   c. hard to change because new mothers feel most comfortable with established routines.
   d. hard to change because most staff are comfortable with established routines.

3. The MOST important reason for an LC to chart information about each contact with a client is to
   a. provide information that is useful to other health-care workers.
   b. avoid legal claims against the LC.
   c. verify the LC's time cards.
   d. substantiate the client's insurance claims.

4. The possibility of a lawsuit brought against an LC can be reduced if certain practices are followed. Which of the following will reduce the likelihood of a lawsuit?

   a. Assume that you have permission to touch the mother and her baby at the outset of each client visit.

   b. Explain what procedures you wish to perform and what information those procedures will elicit, and ask permission to proceed.

   c. Be honest and direct in your discussions with the mother, even if it means making harsh statements.

   d. Reveal the mother and baby's identity if you discuss this case with other LCs.

5. As an LC, you see a mother and young breastfeeding infant for recent poor weight gain. You note that the infant is feverish and listless. What do you do now?

   a. Evaluate recent breastfeeding behavior and suggest ways to stimulate the baby.

   b. Evaluate recent breastfeeding behavior, suggest ways to stimulate the baby, and offer suggestions on how to reduce fever in an infant.

   c. Evaluate recent breastfeeding behavior, suggest ways to stimulate the baby, offer suggestions on how to reduce fever in an infant, and mention the possibility that the baby should be seen by the family's health-care provider.

   d. Refer the mother and baby to the family's health-care provider; assure the mother that you will return to breastfeeding problems after the baby has been evaluated for medical problems.

Discussion Questions

1. Briefly distinguish between a lactation consultant and a voluntary breastfeeding counselor.

2. Define assertiveness as it is used in this chapter. Briefly note how it differs from aggressiveness as a means of reaching a goal or solving a problem.

3. List two advantages and two disadvantages of a solo LC practice as compared with a partnership or group practice.

4. Briefly discuss each of the following legal issues. Include in your discussion an example that clearly avoids the legal problem in question.

   a. permission to touch

   b. avoiding a guarantee

   c. avoiding causing emotional distress

   d. confidentiality of information

5. Outline how in-hospital LCs and private practice LCs can work together to provide complete, long-term services to breastfeeding mothers in the community.

6. Which health-care providers should work together to assist the mother of a breastfeeding baby who has failed to regain birth weight at 1 month of age? What information or skill can each provider best provide? How will the providers communicate with each other to provide optimal care in both the long and short term?

7. What are three sources of didactic or clinical breastfeeding education in your community available to persons who wish to sit the IBLCE exam?

8. Read the discussions of one 24-hour period on an Internet service pertaining to breastfeeding. (If you are not connected to such a service, seek help from a colleague who is.) What does review of these topics tell you about the concerns of LCs today?

9. How do you respond if you are offered a contract to endorse a new nipple cream? Describe the rationale for your response.

ANATOMICAL AND BIOLOGICAL IMPERATIVES

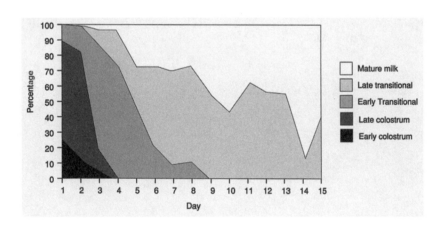

ANATOMY AND PHYSIOLOGY OF LACTATION

Everything we do as lactation consultants is influenced by our understanding of the anatomy of the human breast, the physiology of milk production, the mechanisms of infant suckling, and the responses that drive infant suckling. We must be well grounded in this material before we can thoroughly assess a breastfeeding dyad. Questions in this chapter will help you to assess your understanding of this body of essential information and how it applies to professional practice.

Chapter Outline

Mammogenesis

Breast Structure

Variations

Pregnancy

Lactogenesis

    Delay in lactogenesis

Hormonal Influences

    Progesterone

    Prolactin

    Cortisol

    Thyroid-stimulating hormone (TSH)

    Prolactin-inhibiting factor (PIF)

    Oxytocin

Milk Production

Autocrine versus Endocrine

Galactopoiesis

Multiple-Choice Questions

1. The breasts begin to develop by the fourth week of gestation, when a region of thickened epithelial cells develops that is limited to

   a. two lines that extend from the scapula (shoulder blade) to the groin.

   b. two lines that extend from the axilla (armpit) to the groin.

   c. two lines that extend from the axilla (armpit) to the area underlying the breasts.

   d. the area immediately underlying the breasts.

2. After birth, the newborn's mammary tissue may secrete

   a. a colostrum-like fluid in females but not in males.

   b. a colostrum-like fluid in both males and females.

   c. a plasma-like fluid in males but not in females.

   d. a plasma-like fluid in both males and females.

3. With each menstrual period, the breast continues to add new structures until a woman is about age

   a. 19.   c. 35.

   b. 27.   d. 42.

4. Which of the following statements is FALSE?

   a. A normal breast generally about doubles in weight during lactation.

   b. Breast tissue is anchored to the skin by Cooper's ligaments.

   c. The fourth intercostal nerve is the principal nerve that innervates the nipple and areola.

   d. Mammary ducts widen into sinuses under the areola.

5. A lateral incision at which of the following positions is most likely to sever the nerve that innervates the nipple and areola?

    a. eight o'clock on the right, four o'clock on the left

    b. five o'clock on the right, seven o'clock on the left

    c. ten o'clock on the right, two o'clock on the left

    d. nine o'clock on the right, three o'clock on the left

6. Milk is secreted in alveoli, where it remains until a signal from the hormone _____, produced by the _____ gland, causes _____ cells to contract and force milk into milk ductules.

    a. Oxytocin, posterior pituitary, myoepithelial

    b. Oxytocin, anterior pituitary, squamous cuboidal

    c. Prolactin, posterior pituitary, myoepithelial

    d. Prolactin, anterior pituitary, squamous cuboidal

7. Which of the following statements about breast asymmetry is true?

    a. Breasts almost always are of the same size (symmetrical).

    b. Any breast asymmetry should be considered a marker for problems producing milk.

    c. When breasts are asymmetrical, the right breast usually is larger than the left.

    d. Markedly asymmetrical breasts should be considered a marker for problems producing milk.

8. Accessory nipples and underlying breast tissue

    a. rarely occur except in the groin.

    b. may swell slightly as lactogenesis II occurs but cannot produce milk.

    c. may occur anywhere along the primitive milk line.

    d. almost always develop in pairs.

9. Which statement about nipple protractility (nipple eversion when the base of the nipple shaft is gently compressed) is true?

    a. Nipples tend to be more protractile during a first pregnancy than during subsequent pregnancies.

    b. The degree of nipple protractility increases during a given pregnancy.

    c. About half of all women show poor nipple protractility during their first pregnancy.

    d. Poor nipple protractility is closely related to breastfeeding difficulty.

10. During pregnancy, the

    a. nipples become less erect.

    b. nipples become less protractile.

    c. areolas take on a lighter color.

    d. diameter of the areolas increases.

11. During pregnancy, the breast enlarges under the influence of several hormones. Milk ducts grow and branch under the influence of _____, whereas the lobes, lobules, and alveoli grow under the influence of _____.

    a. estrogen, placental lactogen

    b. estrogen, progesterone

    c. prolactin, progesterone

    d. progesterone, estrogen

12. After a minimum of _____ weeks of pregnancy, a woman's body will produce milk even if the pregnancy ends.

    a. 12

    b. 16

    c. 20

    d. 24

13. Which of the following statements about lactogenesis II is true? It will occur

    a. even if breasts are not stimulated in the first 2 or 3 days postpartum.

    b. only if fluid is actually removed from the breasts by a nursing baby or by a pump in the first 2 or 3 days postpartum.

    c. sooner if breasts are stimulated by a nursing baby or by a pump in the first 2 or 3 days postpartum.

    d. earlier in women who have insulin-dependent diabetes.

14. The capacity of the mammary gland to secrete milk during later pregnancy is called

    a. galactopoiesis.

    b. lactogenesis II.

    c. mammogenesis.

    d. lactogenesis I.

15. Which of the following statements is true about lactogenesis I?

    a. Epithelial cells differentiate into milk secretory cells.

    b. Tight junctions form between secretory cells.

    c. In a normal pregnancy it is complete by month 6.

    d. Breast size increases markedly because milk secretory cells swell with water.

16. After the placenta is delivered, which of the following changes in nutrient concentration take place in the alveoli of the breast?

    a. Sodium and protein decrease, milk fat and lactose increase.

    b. Milk fat and lactose decrease, sodium and protein increase.

    c. Sodium and milk fat decrease, protein and lactose increase.

    d. Protein and lactose decrease, sodium and milk fat increase.

17. After the placenta is delivered, which of the following changes in hormone concentration take place?

    a. Concentrations of progesterone, prolactin, and oxytocin rise.

    b. Concentration of progesterone remain stable, but concentrations of prolactin and oxytocin rise.

   c. Concentrations of progesterone and prolactin fall, but concentration of oxytocin rises.

   d. Concentration of progesterone falls, but concentrations of oxytocin and prolactin rise.

18. Once lactation is initiated, the principle hormone maintaining milk production is

   a. insulin.

   b. dopamine.

   c. prolactin.

   d. oxytocin.

19. During established lactation, the serum concentration of prolactin

   a. is higher at night than in the day.

   b. is closely related to milk yield.

   c. rises shortly after suckling ends at each feeding.

   d. is unrelated to the return of ovulation.

20. Following birth, how is serum prolactin concentration affected by suckling? Assume 10 feeding bouts per 24-hour day.

   a. It peaks with each suckling bout and declines markedly between feeds.

   b. It peaks with each suckling bout and remains near peak levels between feeds.

   c. It gradually drops to baseline and remains there during the first several months of breastfeeding.

   d. It gradually climbs during the first several months of breastfeeding.

21. A secondary effect of oxytocin secretion is

   a. continued milk production.

   b. uterine relaxation.

   c. a slight drop in maternal breast temperature.

   d. heightened maternal anxiety.

22. As compared with a mother who exclusively breastfeeds, a mother who supplements her breastfeeding infant with formula will experience

   a. higher plasma concentrations of oxytocin and prolactin.

   b. lower plasma concentrations of oxytocin and prolactin.

   c. higher plasma concentration of oxytocin, but lower plasma concentration of prolactin.

   d. lower plasma concentration of prolactin, but higher plasma concentration of oxytocin.

23. During the first few days postpartum, frequent suckling should be encouraged, because frequent suckling

   a. is thought to increase the number of prolactin receptors in the breast.

   b. stimulates high levels of progesterone.

   c. speeds up the closure of tight junctions between lactocytes.

   d. is needed to initiate lactogenesis II.

24. Increased skin temperature during a breastfeeding episode is a result of
    a. prolactin secretion.
    b. oxytocin secretion.
    c. cortisol secretion.
    d. TSH secretion.

25. As the number of mammary gland receptors for prolactin _____, breastmilk output _____.
    a. decreases, increases
    b. increases, decreases
    c. decreases, remains the same
    d. increases, increases

26. At birth, an infant's tongue normally occupies what percentage of the oral space when his or her mouth is closed?
    a. about 25 percent
    b. about 50 percent
    c. about 75 percent
    d. nearly 100 percent

27. A newborn will increase suckling activity in response to
    a. sweet taste.
    b. sour taste.
    c. salty taste.
    d. bitter taste.

28. A healthy term infant who has difficulty properly latching onto and milking the breast is most likely to have which of the following conditions?
    a. a palatal arch lacking rugae
    b. buccal fat pads that impinge upon the tongue
    c. a frenulum that is too short or too far forward
    d. cheeks that are too full

29. A suckling reflex in the fetus may be displayed as early as _____ weeks' gestation.
    a. 20   c. 28
    b. 24   d. 32

30. How does a neonate's tongue move with normal suckling at the breast?
    a. in a slight peristaltic motion from back to front
    b. in a slight peristaltic motion from front to back
    c. from side to side as tongue is extended
    d. in a slight motion solely up and down

31. When milk is actively flowing, infants suck and swallow at what average frequency?

    a. twice per second

    b. once per second

    c. once every two seconds

    d. twice every three seconds

32. As milk flow _____, the rate of infant suckling _____.

    a. increases, decreases

    b. decreases, decreases

    c. increases, increases

    d. These variables are unrelated.

33. Active suckling, in addition to providing milk for the infant, also decreases all of the following in the infant EXCEPT

    a. metabolic rate.

    b. feelings of anxiety.

    c. pain threshold.

    d. heart rate.

34. Nonnutritive suckling by premature infants decreases

    a. secretion of digestive fluids.

    b. gastrointestinal peristalsis.

    c. time spent in quiet alert state.

    d. crying.

35. A breastfeeding infant, when properly latched onto the breast, creates

    a. suction that elongates the mother's nipple.

    b. suction that is the principal cause of milk ejection.

    c. suction at initial latch-on that is released as the milk lets down.

    d. no suction.

36. As compared with an infant who is bottle-fed manufactured milk, a breastfed baby

    a. feeds about the same number of times per 24-hour day.

    b. maintains a higher level of oxygen in his or her blood.

    c. has a lower skin temperature.

    d. has a larger requirement for water.

Discussion Questions

1. Discuss the relationship between form and function of the breast in terms of lactational capacity.

2. Describe the form, location, and function in lactation of each of the following structures:
   a. lactiferous duct
   b. adipose cells
   c. milk glands
   d. myoepithelial cells
   e. nipple
   f. areola

3. Explain the relationship between prolactin release, oxytocin release, milk production, and milk ejection.

4. Distinguish between breastfeeding and bottle-feeding in terms of the following:
   a. infant sounds
   b. frequency of suckling
   c. breathing patterns
   d. mouth extension
   e. tongue placement and action
   f. lip flanging
   g. feeding duration

5. "What the baby does is a simple activity, involving negative pressure and swallowing what he or she obtains." Does this statement jibe with current thought? Why or why not?

6. What is meant by the "supply and demand" response of the lactating breast?

7. Explain the relationship between breast size, milk production, and milk storage capacity.

8. Outline a short presentation to a prenatal class on the following topics:
   a. "How the Breast Produces Milk"
   b. "The Baby's Contribution to Successful Breastfeeding"

THE BIOLOGICAL SPECIFICITY OF BREASTMILK

During the long course of mammalian evolution, the milk of each species has acquired properties that meet the nutritional, immunological, and developmental needs of the infants for whom it is the sole nutriment for some period. Because the physical and cognitive abilities of neonates of different species differ widely (consider, for instance, newborn whales, mice, muskox, and humans), so do the constituents of mothers' milk. A thoughtful lactation consultant must understand the basic biology of human milk and how it influences breastfeeding practices. Questions in this chapter will help you assess your knowledge of this essential body of information and how it applies to professional practice.

Chapter Outline

Milk Synthesis and Maturational Changes

Energy, Volume, and Growth

    Caloric density

    Milk volume and storage capacity

    Differences in milk volume between breasts

    Infant growth

Nutritional Values

    Fat

    Lactose

    Protein

    Vitamins and micronutrients

    Minerals

    Preterm milk

Anti-Infective Properties

    Gastroenteritis and diarrheal disease

Multiple-Choice Questions

1. Which of the following does NOT influence breastmilk composition?
   a. gestational age of a newborn
   b. overall duration of lactation
   c. the point (beginning or ending) of a feeding
   d. maternal intake of water-soluble vitamins

2. Compared with mature milk, colostrum is
   a. richer in protein but lower in minerals and carbohydrates.
   b. richer in fats but lower in protein and minerals.
   c. richer in protein and minerals but lower in carbohydrates and fats.
   d. richer in carbohydrates but lower in protein.

3. Approximately how much colostrum does a newborn ingest during the first 24 hours postpartum?

   a. Average, about 11 ml (range, 5–50 ml)

   b. Average, about 38 ml (range, 10–120 ml)

   c. Average, about 74 ml (range, 40–140 ml)

   d. Average, about 100 ml (range, 40–140 ml)

4. After the composition of breast fluid changes from colostrum to mature breastmilk, the total dosage of immunoglobulins received daily by a fully breastfed infant

   a. declines gradually through the sixth month.

   b. declines sharply in transitional milk and then very gradually through the sixth month.

   c. remains approximately constant throughout lactation.

   d. increases steadily through the sixth month.

5. What is the approximate proportion of water to other components in human milk?

   a. 90:10   c. 70:30

   b. 80:20   d. 60:40

6. As compared with manufactured milk, the gastric half-emptying time of breastmilk is

   a. slightly greater for breastmilk.

   b. slightly less for breastmilk.

   c. markedly greater for breastmilk.

   d. markedly less for breastmilk.

7. Does a thriving, fully breastfed infant require added water?

   a. Yes, if the baby lives in a hot, dry climate.

   b. Yes, if the baby lives in a hot, moist climate.

   c. Yes, if the baby is premature.

   d. No, if the baby is normal and healthy.

8. The approximate calorie content of human milk is

   a. 48 kcal/dl.   c. 78 kcal/dl.

   b. 65 kcal/dl.   d. 85 kcal/dl.

9. As compared with breastfed infants, formula-fed infants

   a. do not digest formula very efficiently, so they need a calorie content higher than breastmilk in order to thrive.

   b. tend to be less active, so they need a calorie content lower than breastmilk in order to avoid overfeeding.

   c. have similar calorie requirements, so formula has a calorie content similar to that of breastmilk.

   d. take smaller volumes because they also take supplemental water; thus the calorie density of formula needs to be higher than that of breastmilk.

10. During the first 4 months of life, the nutrient intake of healthy, fully breastfed infants is _____ is currently recommended.

    a. about the same as

    b. about 10 percent greater than

    c. about 10 percent less than

    d. about 20 percent less than

11. When solid foods are added to the diet of a fully breastfed infant, the infant usually

    a. increases her average daily calorie intake.

    b. decreases her average daily calorie intake.

    c. lays down markedly more body fat.

    d. maintains her usual average calorie intake.

12. As compared with infants fed manufactured milk, breastfed infants have

    a. higher energy intake.

    b. lower total daily energy expenditure.

    c. higher heart rate.

    d. higher rectal temperature.

13. What is the approximate average daily volume of milk produced by a mother of a 6-month-old single infant?

    a. 500 ml/day   c. 1000 ml/day

    b. 800 ml/day   d. 1400 ml/day

14. By day five, after lactogenesis II has begun, milk volume averages

    a. 200 ml/day.   c. 900 ml/day.

    b. 500 ml/day.   d. 1300 ml/day.

15. As compared with first-time mothers, multiparous mothers produce _____ milk at 1 week postpartum.

    a. more

    b. less

    c. about the same amount of

    d. more calorie-dense

16. As compared with breastmilk produced by women in their thirties, the breastmilk of adolescent mothers

    a. contains fewer calories.

    b. contains a larger proportion of proteins.

    c. is of smaller daily volume.

    d. is about the same.

17. Large-breasted women

    a. generally produce less milk per day than small-breasted women.

    b. can store larger volumes of milk than small-breasted women.

c. generally feed more often per 24 hours than small-breasted women.

d. must feed at more regular intervals than small-breasted women.

18. The capacity of the breast to synthesize milk normally

    a. just barely meets the infant's need.

    b. generally exceeds the infant's need.

    c. meets the infant's need during the early months, but falls below the infant's need by about 4 months.

    d. meets the infant's need during the early months, but falls below the infant's need by about 6 months.

19. Studies of breast-volume changes ("breast storage capacity") during lactation show that

    a. only large-breasted women usually make more milk than their infants need for adequate growth.

    b. the ability to adequately nourish an infant at the breast diminishes as breast size diminishes.

    c. the amount of milk produced in a 24-hour period is not related to breast size.

    d. storage capacity can be increased by increasing the interval between feedings.

20. The rate of milk synthesis

    a. is about the same in both breasts during a given woman's course of lactation.

    b. is generally greater in the left breast than in the right.

    c. depends on the degree of emptying of the breast.

    d. is more rapid in the first few weeks but slows as breastfeeding becomes established.

21. The rate of milk synthesis

    a. varies within narrow limits for a given woman.

    b. is fixed at a lower level in primiparas than in multiparas.

    c. is controlled by systemic hormonal signals originating in the brain.

    d. varies within wide limits among women in general.

22 The amount of breastmilk that an infant will ingest during the entire course of lactation is most closely correlated with

    a. maternal parity.

    b. maternal weight gain during pregnancy.

    c. infant birth weight.

    d. infant weight at 1 month.

23. What pattern of weight gain typifies a fully breastfed infant?

    a. a steady rate of weight gain (5 to 7 oz/week) through the first 6 months

    b. rapid gain in the first month (average 5 to 7 oz/week) followed by decreasing rate of weight gain through the sixth month

    c. an initial rate of weight gain at about 3 oz/week that increases through the sixth month

    d. rapid gain until about the fourth month, then a rapid decline in rate of weight gain until solids are started

24. Breastfed infants need _____ than artificially fed babies to grow adequately.

    a. more kcal/unit of body weight

    b. more kcal/unit of body weight after 5 months of age than before 5 months of age

    c. much longer feedings

    d. fewer kcal/unit of body weight

25. Which of the following statements about fats in breastmilk is NOT true?

    a. The enzyme lipase, which breaks down milk fats, is found only in the intestines.

    b. The fat content of normal breastmilk provides about half of the milk's calories.

    c. The early milk of preterm mothers contains considerably more fat than the milk of mothers who deliver at term.

    d. Triglycerides are the main fats in breastmilk.

26. With respect to the fat content of human milk, maternal dietary fat intake

    a. does influence the total amount, but not the type of fats.

    b. does not influence the total amount, but does influence the types of fat.

    c. does influence both the amount and types of fat present.

    d. does not influence either the amount or the types of fat present.

27. During a given feeding, the fat concentration of human milk

    a. is remarkably stable throughout.

    b. is inversely related to the degree to which the breast is emptied.

    c. is higher the longer the interval since the last feeding.

    d. is directly related to the degree to which the breast is emptied at that feeding.

28. The BEST way to increase the amount of fat ingested by a baby during one breastfeeding is to encourage the baby to

    a. feed on both breasts at each feeding.

    b. feed on only one breast at each feeding.

    c. switch back and forth between breasts several times.

    d. feed at longer intervals than usual.

29 Lactose intolerance

    a. is common in formula-fed infants.

    b. is caused by the presence of lactase in the intestinal mucosa.

    c. develops progressively after weaning.

    d. refers to the baby's inability to synthesize lactose.

30. Which of the following statements about the whey and casein composition of human milk is true?

    a. Whey forms tough, less digestible curds than does casein.

    b. Casein is usually present in equal or greater concentration than whey.

c. Whey is usually present in equal or greater concentration than casein.

d. The ratio of whey to casein is fixed for the course of lactation.

31. Which of the following situations produces higher than usual sodium levels in breastmilk?

a. onset of lactogenesis II

b. suddenly increased frequency of nursing ("growth spurts")

c. allergic reactions in the mother such as hay-fever

d. weaning

32. As compared with mature breastmilk, colostrum contains

a. a higher concentration of lactose.

b. a lower concentration of protein.

c. lower concentrations of IgA and lactoferrin.

d. higher concentrations of the essential amino acids.

33. Breastfed children at lowest risk of developing rickets are those

a. who are dark skinned.

b. who regularly use sunscreen and wear sun-protective clothing.

c. whose skin is regularly exposed to small doses of sun.

d. whose mothers consume a vegan (no animal products) diet.

34. Infants whose mothers consume a vegan diet (without meat or dairy) during pregnancy may be more susceptible to the development of

a. undescended testicles in males.

b. extremely fair and fragile skin.

c. inner-ear problems leading to poor balance.

d. neural tube defects.

35. High pharmacologic dosages of vitamin B_6 given to a breastfeeding mother have been found to

a. increase the rate of prolactin secretion.

b. cause neurological problems in breastfed infants.

c. decrease the rate of prolactin secretion.

d. ameliorate neurological problems in breastfed infants.

36. Adding iron to an otherwise fully breastfed infant's diet

a. is essential during months two through six to ensure adequate brain growth.

b. impairs the effectiveness of the anti-infective agent lactoferrin.

c. is not necessary because breastmilk contains a high concentration of iron.

d. promotes the effectiveness of the anti-infective agent lactoferrin.

37. In their first several months, healthy breastfed infants rarely need iron supplements

a. because lactose and vitamin C in breastmilk facilitate absorption of iron.

b. because breastmilk is naturally high in iron.

    c. if the mother herself regularly ingests an iron supplement.

    d. with the exception of infants of vegetarian mothers.

38. Compared with the early milk of mothers who deliver term infants, the early milk of mothers who deliver preterm infants contains

    a. lower concentrations of calories.

    b. higher concentrations of proteins.

    c. lower concentrations of anti-inflammatory factors.

    d. higher concentrations of all vitamins.

39. A child who is not breastfed is at greater risk for

    a. acute illnesses, but not chronic illnesses.

    b. chronic illnesses, but not acute illnesses.

    c. both acute and chronic illnesses.

    d. neither acute nor chronic illnesses.

40. The most important way that exclusive breastfeeding for at least 6 months mitigates allergic responses is by

    a. allowing time for IgE to lay down a protective coating on intestinal mucosa.

    b. facilitating the early maturation of an intestinal barrier to lactoferrin.

    c. minimizing exposure of the baby's gut to foreign proteins.

    d. promoting binding of potential allergens on the intestinal mucosa.

41. Breastmilk influences an infant's immune response by

    a. conferring passive immunity that persists into early childhood.

    b. stimulating an active immune response.

    c. increasing the infant's white cell count as long as he continues to breastfeed.

    d. erasing the immune system's long-term memory.

42. Secretory IgA is

    a. manufactured by the placenta and stored in the breast.

    b. the most widely active immunoglobulin in human secretions.

    c. present in lower concentrations in mothers whose infants have chronic infections.

    d. ingested in markedly smaller dosages from breastmilk than from colostrum.

43. The intestinal environment of the fully breastfed infant discourages the proliferation of coliform bacteria because

    a. gram-positive lactobacilli and *L. bifidus* are only minor fecal flora.

    b. it discourages the growth of a lactobacilli-promoting factor.

    c. factors in breastmilk sequester coliform bacteria by promoting their adhesion to the intestinal wall.

    d. it has a low pH (i.e., it is acid).

Discussion Questions

1. Why is human milk sometimes referred to as "white blood"?

2. How does each of the following factors affect breastmilk composition and volume?

    a. the gestational age of the infant

    b. the mother's age

    c. the beginning of the feed

    d. the end of the feed

    e. the preterm baby's gestational age

3. It has been reported that breastfed infants, as compared with infants fed manufactured milks, consume approximately 30,000 fewer kcal by 8 months of age. Of what significance to the individual baby is this finding? Of what significance to overall infant health?

4. Briefly discuss the role of human milk in reducing infant morbidity and mortality resulting from

    a. diarrhea.

    b. gastrointestinal infections.

    c. upper respiratory infections.

5. What is the "bifidus factor" and how does it protect the breastfeeding infant's gut?

6. What is the relationship between lactoferrin and iron? What is the mechanism by which exogenous iron may reduce lactoferrin's capacity to function?

7. By what mechanisms does breastmilk reduce the likelihood of an allergic reaction in an infant? Explain at least four mechanisms.

8. What is the primary nutritional role of each of the following compounds? How do suboptimal amounts of each affect infant health?

    a. fat

    b. fat-soluble vitamins

    c. iron

    d. protein

    e. water-soluble vitamins

    f. zinc

9. What is the relationship between the concentration of immunoglobulins in colostrum and in mature breastmilk? From which secretion does the infant obtain the greatest volume of immunoglobulins?

10. Taurine has been added to some manufactured baby milks. Do you think the effectiveness of taurine is the same in manufactured milks as in breastmilk? Why or why not?

11. Given 30 minutes to talk, what three main points would you make about human milk to

    a. physician assistant students, who need clinically important information?

    b. medical students, who want to know all the biochemistry as well as clinically important information?

5

Drug Therapy and Breastfeeding

Mother is ill; baby is breastfeeding. Where is the balance point between treating the mother and perhaps forgoing breastfeeding, or maintaining breastfeeding and perhaps risking the mother's health? A firm grounding in the pharmacokinetics of drug uptake into milk, the concentration of drug that reaches the infant, and how an infant metabolizes the drug will help the lactation consultant judge the risks involved. Questions in this chapter will help you to assess your understanding of this body of knowledge and how it applies to professional practice.

Chapter Outline

Multiple-Choice Questions

1. Which of the following statements is true?
   a. Most but not all drugs pass into human milk in concentrations of clinical concern.
   b. Most medications appear in low, subclinical amounts in human milk.
   c. Most drugs are contraindicated in the breastfeeding mother.
   d. If a drug is taken by mouth, the drug does not reach the baby because it is destroyed in the mother's stomach.

2. To calculate the dosage of a maternal drug that is ingested by a breastfeeding infant, one must know
   a. the concentration of drug in maternal plasma.
   b. the concentration of drug in foremilk.
   c. the concentration of drug in hindmilk.
   d. the concentration of drug in breastmilk as a whole.

3. The transfer of most drugs into human milk involves which of the following?
   a. active transport
   b. a concentration gradient
   c. ionized or bound compounds
   d. an impermeable membrane

4. Which of the following promotes a given drug's transfer into human milk?

    a. low levels in maternal plasma

    b. greater tendency to bind to proteins

    c. lower molecular weight

    d. lesser tendency to dissolve in fats

5. The proportion of a drug transferred from mother to a breastfeeding infant during the first 2 or 3 days postpartum is most likely to be

    a. large, because lactocytes (cells lining the mammary alveoli) are small.

    b. small, because diffusion is working at low efficiency.

    c. large, because protein-bound drugs are more likely to appear in colostrum.

    d. small, because the amount of colostrum ingested is small.

6. The best way to minimize transfer of maternal medications to a breastfeeding infant is to use medications that have a

    a. long half-life and are taken right after a feeding.

    b. short half-life and are taken right after a feeding.

    c. long half-life and are taken right before a feeding.

    d. short half-life and are taken right before a feeding.

7. Which of the following statements about a drug's milk/plasma ratio (the ratio of concentrations of a drug in milk and in maternal plasma) is true?

    a. Drugs with a high milk/plasma ratio are transferred to the infant in high dosages.

    b. High milk/plasma ratios may or may not result in high concentrations of drug in the infant.

    c. Maternal plasma concentration is less important than milk/plasma ratio in determining milk concentration.

    d. The volume of milk ingested by the infant exerts little control on the infant's dose.

8. The concentration of a drug in maternal plasma depends on all of the following EXCEPT

    a. the dose administered.

    b. the half-life of the drug.

    c. the drug's lipid solubility.

    d. the bioavailability of drugs taken by mouth.

9. The amount of a drug transferred to an infant through breastmilk is increased if

    a. the volume of breastmilk ingested is small.

    b. the drug has low oral bioavailability in the mother.

    c. the drug has high oral bioavailability in the infant.

    d. maternal plasma concentrations are low.

10. The greatest amount of maternal medication is transferred to a

    a. 3-month-old infant who is taking close to 1 liter/day of mother's milk.

    b. 1- to 3-month-old infant who is nursing at least 8 times in 24 hours.

    c. 4-day-old neonate who is breastfeeding but not yet stooling very often.

    d. fetus still linked by a placenta to her mother.

11. A medication used by a breastfeeding mother should have an oral bioavailability that is

    a. high, so individual dosages can be small.

    b. high, so that the greatest amount passes into maternal plasma.

    c. low, so that it will be degraded in her stomach or intestines.

    d. low, so that it will be degraded in the infant's stomach or intestines.

12. The infant dosage of a drug administered to a breastfeeding mother is apt to be highest if the drug is

    a. just barely detectable in maternal plasma.

    b. applied topically (e.g., steroids, antibiotics).

    c. given as a single injection (e.g., anesthetics).

    d. given as several sequenced injections.

13. As compared with a 4-month-old infant, the risk to a 12-month-old infant of drugs in breastmilk is

    a. greater because the older infant is likely taking solids as well as breastmilk.

    b. lower because the older infant takes a smaller volume of milk per unit of body weight.

    c. greater because the younger infant's immune system is less likely to be stressed.

    d. lower because the younger infant will ingest a smaller volume of breastmilk.

14. To minimize possible harm to her breastfeeding infant, a mother who must take a medication should avoid which of the following practices?

    a. feeding stored breastmilk during the interval that the mother must use a medication

    b. using a maternal medication that is considered safe for use in young children

    c. using medications with lower protein-binding capacity

    d. using higher molecular weight medications

15. Estrogen and progesterone, singly or in combination (the constituents) of contraceptive pills,

    a. may reduce breastmilk supply, especially if they are used during the first few weeks postpartum.

    b. may increase milk supply if use is delayed until the baby is at least 4 months old.

    c. are best begun in the immediate postpartum when maternal hormone levels are still in flux.

    d. are unlikely to reduce milk supply if the baby is several months old when the mother begins taking them.

16. Bromocriptine, which was once widely used to inhibit breastmilk production, is

    a. still the drug of choice for reducing engorgement and inhibiting milk production.

    b. still the drug of choice for inhibiting breastmilk production, but not for reducing engorgement.

    c. no longer recommended because it is associated with serious cardiac problems.

    d. no longer recommended because it is associated with gastrointestinal perforation.

17. Compounds such as metoclopramide and domperidone, which can increase prolactin levels, are MOST appropriately used in mothers

    a. whose prolactin levels are low, such as some mothers of premature infants.

    b. of all premature infants in dosages that raise prolactin concentration to very high levels.

    c. of healthy term infants when the mothers' milk supply is low.

    d. of healthy term infants when the mothers must return to work.

18. The mother of a young breastfed infant tells you that she is drinking fenugreek tea. What is her most likely reason?

    a. She likes the taste of fenugreek.

    b. Fenugreek is known to dry up mother's milk without causing pain.

    c. It is known be a topical analgesic.

    d. It is thought to be a galactagogue.

19. Mothers who use penicillins or cephalosporins have been shown to produce breastmilk that is

    a. high in both penicillins and cephalosporins.

    b. low in both penicillins and cephalosporins.

    c. high in penicillins but low in cephalosporins.

    d. high in cephalosporins but low in penicillins.

20. When a mother must take a medication, that drug's effect on the infant can be minimized by

    a. using a medication that is considered safe for treating infants.

    b. breastfeeding when the medication is at higher concentration in the mother's plasma.

    c. using a medication with a longer half-life.

    d. using a medication that has higher oral bioavailability.

21. Drugs that enter the central nervous system

    a. are likely to enter breastmilk.

    b. are unlikely to enter breastmilk.

    c. are typically of low molecular weight and bind easily to protein.

    d. are typically of high molecular weight and very lipid soluble.

22. As compared with full-term infants, preterm infants

    a. have similar responses to medications.

    b. require higher dosages to achieve the same therapeutic effect.

    c. typically clear medications from the body more slowly, which causes more adverse reactions.

    d. typically bind drugs less effectively, which lessens their effect on the infant.

Discussion Questions

1. What characteristics regulate the passage of molecules into breastmilk?

2. Describe at least three reliable sources of information about drug use during lactation.

3. What are at least four strategies for reducing a breastfeeding infant's exposure to a medication ingested by his mother?

4. Would you be concerned about the effects on her 2-day-old infant from a sleep medication used by a new mother? Why or why not? Would your degree of concern for the infant be the same if the mother used the same medication 2 months later? Why or why not?

5. A breastfeeding mother with a 2-week-old baby asks you if she should continue to take pain pills intended to relieve the pain following a cesarean section. What do you tell this mother? What is your rationale?

6. A mother presents with nipples that are red and extremely painful. She has been taking an antibiotic for a month since her cesarean section. What do you suspect to be the culprit? Why? What do you recommend?

7. Can a mother of a 6-week-old breastfeeding infant use a bronchodilator containing ephedrine to control asthma? What do you tell the mother? What is your rationale?

8. Do topical agents, such as those used to reduce the discomfort of poison ivy, appear in breastmilk in clinical amounts? If the nursing baby has begun solids already, is it better to use the topical agent and wean the baby? Why or why not?

VIRUSES AND BREASTFEEDING

Because human milk is a highly cellular fluid, it transmits viruses (which reproduce inside cells); however, it also transmits antibodies that help the infant resist those viruses. A lactation consultant must understand the natural history of transmission of viruses from mother to child and how the modes of transmission and effect on the infant differ in the pregnant and the breastfeeding mother. Questions in this chapter will help you to assess your understanding of this body of information and how it applies to professional practice.

Chapter Outline

Key Concepts

Internet Resources

References

Multiple-Choice Questions

1. The passive immunity to childhood diseases that is received by breastfed infants persists
   a. for about 3 to 6 weeks.
   b. for about 3 to 6 months.
   c. during the period of exclusive breastfeeding.
   d. during the period in which any breastmilk is ingested.

2. Viruses can be transmitted between mother and infant during breastfeeding because
   a. of the close physical contact between mother and infant.
   b. breastmilk is mostly water, in which viruses are soluble.
   c. breastmilk is unable to inactivate the viruses it may contain.
   d. breastmilk contains many cells, in which viruses live.

3. According to a 1999 study, exclusive breastfeeding appears to offer some protection against HIV transmission to infants in third world areas PRIMARILY because it
   a. confers immunologic protection.
   b. contains vitamin A.
   c. protects the infant's intestinal mucosal barrier.
   d. avoids contamination from early solid foods.

4. When a baby is born to a mother infected with HIV, the risk of transmission of the virus through breastmilk is
   a. negligible as compared with the fetal transmission rate.
   b. about 50 percent higher than the fetal transmission rate.
   c. about 10 to 15 percent greater than the fetal transmission rate.
   d. highest in women in industrialized countries.

5. Universal precautions designed to protect health-care workers against infection through contact with patients apply to
   a. blood, human milk, and semen.
   b. human milk, semen, and vaginal secretions.
   c. semen, vaginal secretions, and blood.
   d. vaginal secretions, human milk, and blood.

6. A woman who receives a diagnosis of primary chickenpox within a week before or within 2 days after delivery should be
   a. allowed to initiate breastfeeding as usual.
   b. retained in hospital for at least 4 days.

    c. isolated with her infant in all cases.

    d. isolated with her infant only if the infant also has chickenpox lesions.

7. To ensure the safety of an infant born to a pregnant woman infected with herpes simplex virus, vaginal delivery is

    a. always contraindicated.

    b. contraindicated if active genital lesions are present at delivery.

    c. contraindicated if the mother acquired her virus infection during this pregnancy.

    d. contraindicated if the mother acquired the virus some time before this pregnancy.

8. The most common path by which herpes virus is thought to be transmitted between mother and infant during breastfeeding is

    a. virus contained in the milk.

    b. infant contact with active lesions on the mother's breast.

    c. inhalation by the baby of expired maternal air that contains virus in respiratory droplets.

    d. ungloved maternal hands that hold the infant for a feeding.

9. A herpes simplex virus infection is most likely to harm the infant of a mother first infected with this virus when the infant

    a. is a newborn.

    b. is about 6 months old and is taking maximal amounts of breastmilk.

    c. has recently weaned completely from the breast.

    d. is of any age; age has nothing to do with the seriousness of this infection.

10. A mother who contracts viral illnesses such as varicella zoster (chickenpox), rubella, or cytomegalovirus while she is breastfeeding a 4-month-old infant should

    a. continue breastfeeding, because these viruses are not passed through breastmilk.

    b. continue breastfeeding, because antibodies to these viruses in breastmilk will help protect the infant.

    c. discontinue breastfeeding, because of the risk of severe illness in her infant.

    d. discontinue breastfeeding, because of the risk of endangering her own health.

11. Which of the following viruses is most prevalent in the adult population?

    a. herpes simplex   c. rubella

    b. toxoplasmosis   d. cytomegalovirus

12. Infants born to women with a history of hepatitis B virus

    a. should breastfeed, because infants not breastfed are more likely to contract the disease.

    b. should not breastfeed, because breastfed infants of infected mothers have a higher rate of hepatitis B infection.

    c. should breastfeed, because breastfeeding lowers the mother's plasma concentration of this virus.

    d. should not breastfeed, because virus in breastmilk stresses the infant's immature liver.

13. Which of the following viruses is usually considered to contraindicate breastfeeding?

    a. rubella
    b. hepatitis B
    c. HTLV-1
    d. herpes simplex

Discussion Questions

1. Where do viruses replicate? How does this site influence the modes of transmission of viral illnesses?

2. Under what circumstances might a mother with herpes zoster continue to breastfeed her infant?

3. How is it that rubella can cause birth defects, but is of no concern if it appears in breastmilk?

4. Does breastfeeding appear to increase the risk of hepatitis B infection in infants? What is the rationale for your answer?

5. Should a mother with a known viral infection (not HIV) breastfeed her newborn? What is the rationale for your response?

6. What is "passive immunity"?

7. What are current recommendations about whether a mother with HIV should breastfeed? What considerations govern those recommendations?

8. How does the relative timing of a woman's initial HIV infection and the index pregnancy (the pregnancy being evaluated now) affect the risk of transmission to the infant? When is the risk of transmission highest? lowest?

9. Create a table with the following headings: Column heads–Route of Transmission, Likelihood of Neonatal Infection, Acute or Chronic Infection, Prevention of Cross-Contamination. Row heads–Herpes Simplex, Cytomegalovirus, Herpes Zoster, Hepatitis B, Hepatitis C, HTLV-1, Rubella. Evaluate the ways in which the viruses are similar and the ways in which they differ.

10. On the basis of the chart created in question 9, draw some conclusions about the advisability of breastfeeding by a mother who has a viral infection. Does the age of the infant make a difference?

11. Compare hepatitis B and hepatitis C with regard to

    a. likelihood of transmission to the fetus.

    b. likelihood of transmission through breastfeeding.

    c. whether breastfeeding should be initiated or (depending on the circumstances) continued.

    d. potential for protection of the child later in life.

    e. potential for later chronic illnesses as a result of exposure to the virus as a fetus or newborn.

12. Should a mother with an episode of active herpes at the time she delivers breastfeed her newborn? Should she room-in with her infant?

13. What precautions should a lactation consultant take when she assists an HIV mother who is experiencing breast engorgement?

14. Should a mother who contracts chickenpox while breastfeeding wean her infant? What is the rationale for your answer?

Prenatal, Perinatal, and Postnatal Periods

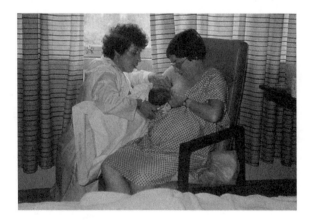

PERINATAL AND INTRAPARTUM CARE

Breastfeeding cannot continue unless it is successfully begun. Thus, how to help a mother and her new baby initiate breastfeeding, whether in normal or in difficult circumstances, is of primary importance. Questions in this chapter will help you to assess your understanding of this body of information and how it applies to professional practice.

Chapter Outline

Multiple-Choice Questions

1. How do you respond to a question about rubbing the nipples and areola with a towel to prepare the nipples for breastfeeding?

   a. It is unnecessary.

   b. It is appropriate if the mother is extremely gentle.

   c. A burning sensation means that the technique is working.

   d. It is necessary only if the mother has very pale or freckled skin.

2. Breastfeeding during the first hour after birth

   a. is generally recommended, because a neonate's suckling reflex is usually strong at this time.

   b. is not generally recommended, because colostrum hasn't developed its full immunological capacity.

   c. is generally recommended, because digestive peristalsis is promoted in the mother, thereby making breastmilk jaundice less likely.

   d. is generally not recommended, because suckling promotes uterine cramping, which increases the loss of blood from the uterus.

3. Epidural analgesia during labor has been associated with

   a. early neonatal suckling and increased suckling vigor.

   b. delayed neonatal suckling and reduced suckling vigor.

   c. early neonatal suckling but reduced suckling vigor.

   d. delayed neonatal suckling but increased suckling vigor.

4. "Clearing the airway" by suctioning the neonate's nose is

   a. recommended, because essentially all neonates are congested at birth.

   b. not recommended, because suctioning may cause congestion.

    c. recommended because, although it may not always be necessary, it can do no harm.

    d. not recommended because the baby may imprint on a firm bulb syringe.

5. During the first 24 hours postpartum, the BEST time to initiate breastfeeding is likely to be

    a. within 2 hours after birth.

    b. around 6 hours after birth.

    c. around 12 hours after birth.

    d. around 24 hours after birth.

6. A neonate spends most of the first 24 hours after birth in which state?

    a. awake, alert

    b. light sleep

    c. deep sleep

    d. light and deep sleep

7. A newborn's licking or nuzzling of his mother's nipples shortly after birth

    a. promotes relaxation of the mother's uterus.

    b. colonizes the baby with the mother's skin flora.

    c. makes the infant more susceptible to pathogenic bacteria.

    d. promotes secretion of witch's milk.

8. Epidural anesthesia or analgesia

    a. has no known effects on the breastfeeding newborn.

    b. may shorten the interval before the baby breastfeeds effectively

    c. may lengthen the interval before the baby breastfeeds effectively

    d. may reduce suckling vigor but does not affect the interval before effective breastfeeds begin.

9. While the baby is learning to latch onto the breast, the BEST moment to bring him to the breast is when

    a. his feet are pressed against the mother's opposite arm, for increased stability.

    b. his eyes are closed, signaling concentration.

    c. his neck, shoulder, and torso are aligned.

    d. his mouth is wide open.

10. During early breastfeedings, the mother should breastfeed a neonate

    a. only on one breast.

    b. on one or both breasts at the baby's discretion.

    c. for no longer than 10 minutes on the first breast or 20 minutes on the second breast.

    d. for no longer than 20 minutes on the first breast but as long as the baby desires on the second.

11. During hand expression, the mother places her fingers an inch or so behind the nipple, and presses gently _____ toward the chest wall, with a slight _____ action toward the nipple.

    a. upward, rolling

    b. downward, rubbing

    c. inward, rubbing

    d. inward, rolling

12. Before attempting to feed a baby who is actively crying, the mother should

    a. change the baby's diaper.

    b. gently hold and console the baby.

    c. ready a supplemental bottle in case the baby feeds poorly at the breast.

    d. distract the baby with rattles or other toys.

13. A baby who is wiggling or moving her hands to her mouth

    a. is tired of her position in a crib or in someone's lap.

    b. needs nonnutritive sucking as a calming device.

    c. is ready to breastfeed.

    d. most likely is trying to protect her eyes from bright light.

14. As the mother's nipple lightly strokes the center of a baby's lower lip, the baby usually opens his mouth widely and

    a. turns his face away.

    b. sneezes.

    c. extends his tongue.

    d. uses his tongue to block the back of his mouth.

15. Which of the following is the LEAST acceptable method of feeding an infant who latches onto the breast poorly during early attempts to feed?

    a. teaspoon

    b. medicine cup

    c. feeding bottle

    d. finger (tube) feeding

16. A healthy 3-week-old 10-pound infant needs to ingest about how many ounces of breastmilk in 24 hours?

    a. 8   c. 24

    b. 16   d. 32

17. Which of the following increases an infant's difficulty in achieving a secure latch onto the breast?

    a. an intact palate

    b. a tongue that is firmly anchored by the frenulum

    c. a tongue that cups up at the edges

    d. a mouth that is comfortable (not sore)

18. When a mother of a newborn who is not feeding well uses a silicone nipple shield, the mother should also
    a. pump her breasts when they feel overly full.
    b. give water by finger-feeding.
    c. check the baby's diapers for adequate urine and stools.
    d. weigh the baby at 2-week intervals.

19. Blood glucose concentrations in breastfed infants are generally
    a. higher than in formula-fed infants.
    b. lower than in bottle-fed infants.
    c. stable in the immediate postpartum period.
    d. inversely correlated with the number of breastfeedings.

20. Which of the following conditions is LEAST likely to lead to hypoglycemia in a newborn infant?
    a. maternal diabetes
    b. maternal hypertension
    c. large for gestational age infant
    d. small for gestational age infant

21. The risk of hypoglycemia in a newborn can be minimized by
    a. loosely wrapping the infant so air can circulate around him.
    b. initiating breastfeeding within the first 2 hours after birth.
    c. initiating breastfeeding about 20 hours after birth, when the infant rouses from a period of deep sleep.
    d. feeding for fixed time periods at regular intervals.

22. As compared with mothers who give birth vaginally, mothers who give birth by cesarean section are
    a. less likely to breastfeed even though lactogenesis II is not delayed.
    b. about as likely to breastfeed but generally breastfeed for fewer months.
    c. less likely to breastfeed but breastfeed for about the same average number of months.
    d. about as likely to breastfeed but have delayed lactogenesis II.

23. Mothers who deliver by cesarean section and who intend to breastfeed benefit MOST from
    a. minimal analgesics for postpartum pain.
    b. delaying initiation of breastfeeding until they are more comfortable.
    c. using standard cradle position for the baby at the breast.
    d. early initiation of breastfeeding.

24. Because a baby born by cesarean section may not latch onto the breast well in the early postpartum, which is the BEST action to take?
    a. Delay first breastfeeding until baby clears maternal analgesia or anesthesia from his system.
    b. Put the baby to breast in the first few hours after birth.

    c. Encourage the mother to immediately begin pumping her breasts to hasten lactogenesis II.

    d. Encourage the mother to immediately begin pumping her breasts to improve later milk transfer.

25. The likelihood of excessive breast engorgement is increased in the mother who

    a. avoids supplements of manufactured milk.

    b. initiates breastfeeding in the early postpartum.

    c. feeds about 8 to 12 times in 24 hours.

    d. ensures that the baby feeds from both breasts at each feeding.

26. In the early weeks, the most reliable indicator that the baby is taking in sufficient milk is

    a. baby's swallows are audible during much of the feeding.

    b. baby wakes on her own for feedings.

    c. baby has several heavy wet diapers and stools each day.

    d. baby gains about 1 to 2 ounces per day.

27. Breastfeeding should be evaluated if the neonate produces

    a. yellowish stools after lactogenesis II is established.

    b. sticky black or green stools before lactogenesis II is established.

    c. red stains or "dust" in the diaper after lactogenesis II is established.

    d. colorless urine at any time.

28. During their first 48 hours of life, and as compared with babies fed artificial milk, exclusively breast-fed infants ingest

    a. a smaller amount of fluid.

    b. a larger amount of fluid.

    c. on average about the same amount of fluid.

    d. less fluid in the first 24 hours but more in the second 24 hours.

29. During normal postpartum engorgement

    a. breast tissue becomes incompressible.

    b. the breast should be offered at as long intervals as the baby will tolerate.

    c. the baby cannot latch onto the breast.

    d. the mother may run a low fever.

30. Before discharge, first-time breastfeeding mothers should be taught all of the following EXCEPT

    a. how to prepare emergency bottles of manufactured milks.

    b. infant feeding cues.

    c. signs of sufficient intake by the baby.

    d. how to latch the baby onto the breast.

31. Recent research has shown that maternity-ward discharge packages containing manufactured milks
    a. do not affect the duration of exclusive breastfeeding.
    b. lengthen the duration of exclusive breastfeeding.
    c. shorten the duration of any breastfeeding.
    d. do not affect the duration of breastfeeding combined with supplemental foods.

Discussion Questions

1. How can a pregnant woman prepare herself for breastfeeding? Describe at least three ways.

2. Describe at least five faulty assumptions about breastfeeding. What is a better way to explain how breastfeeding can work in each situation?

3. Describe at least three different ways to hold a baby for breastfeeding. When is each position best used? What are cautions that apply to each position?

4. What is hypoglycemia? When it is most likely to occur in a neonate? How should the baby be managed? What is the rationale for this management?

5. In a healthy newborn who displays a normal suckling pattern:
    a. what do the baby's cheeks look like?
    b. where is the baby's tongue? Is any of it visible?
    c. what do you hear during suckling bursts?
    d. what do the baby's lips look like?
    e. how firmly is the baby attached to the breast?

6. What is finger-feeding? What are indications for its use? What are cautions about its use?

7. Describe at least three practices in the early postpartum that contribute to breast engorgement in a breastfeeding mother, and then describe better practices that minimize engorgement.

8. Under what circumstances might you use a thin silicone nipple shield to assist breastfeeding? What are cautions about its use?

9. Why does early, frequent breastfeeding promote optimal functioning in both mother and newborn? Discuss at least four reasons, and show how each reason supports the other reasons you discuss.

10. How is postpartum "breast fullness" distinguished from "breast engorgement"? How is each best treated?

Postpartum Care

The information in this chapter expands on that in the preceding chapter and extends into the mother's "fourth trimester." Hallmarks of successful breastfeeding are a confident, comfortable mother and a thriving infant. Questions in this chapter will help you to assess your understanding of how to help mothers and babies achieve these goals.

Chapter Outline

Multiple-Choice Questions

1. According to the American Academy of Pediatrics, the new breastfeeding mother–infant dyad should not be discharged before
   a. the mother decides to go home.
   b. at least two breastfeedings have demonstrated coordinated suckling, swallowing, and breathing.
   c. the baby has roused from his first long sleep on day 1.
   d. at least two feedings of any type have demonstrated coordinated suckling, swallowing, and breathing.

2. Insufficient milk supply
   a. is a real physical problem that occurs in a large percentage of primiparous mothers.
   b. can be resolved most rapidly if the mother supplements the baby for the first 2 weeks of life.
   c. is usually a marker for the lack of desire to breastfeed.
   d. is commonly a conclusion based on misinterpretation of normal infant breastfeeding behavior.

3. When a baby refuses to feed on one breast but will go to the other, the mother
   a. should offer only the less-preferred breast.
   b. will need to use formula supplement to assure adequate infant growth.
   c. should express milk from the less-preferred breast.
   d. wait until the baby is very hungry, to increase the likelihood that she will feed from both breasts.

4. A 2-week-old baby who is alert, cues for feeds, and is content afterwards is apt also to
   a. have firm, elastic skin.
   b. pass no more than one or two soft yellow stools per day.
   c. have more than one long stretch (3 or 4 hours) of deep sleep per 24-hour day.
   d. latch so tightly to the breast that no swallowing is heard.

5. Massage of the lactating breast, a common practice in many cultures, is thought to
   a. decrease lymphatic drainage.
   b. reduce or eliminate intraductal cysts.
   c. increase milk production.
   d. be contraindicated during breast engorgement.

6. When would transitory nipple soreness be most noticeable?
   a. between the first and second postpartum day
   b. between the third and sixth postpartum day
   c. between the sixth and tenth postpartum day
   d. any time in the first 2 weeks.

7. One of the top priorities for discharge teaching for breastfeeding families is
   a. to feed the baby on cue around the clock.
   b. the best type of clothing to wear for discreet breastfeeding.
   c. where the mother can obtain a breast pump.
   d. coping with a crying baby.

8. Of the treatments listed below, which pair best relieves nipple soreness while posing the least risk to mother or infant?
   a. purified lanolin, antibiotic cream
   b. purified lanolin, warm water
   c. breastmilk, warm water
   d. tea bags, antiseptics

9. A healthy term neonate will regain her birth weight no later than _____ postpartum.
   a. 5 days   c. 2 weeks
   b. 1 week   d. 3 weeks

10. A thriving, 2-month-old, exclusively breastfed infant can be expected to gain about 4 to 7 ounces
    a. per day.   c. per 2 weeks.
    b. per week.   d. per month.

11. The effectiveness of breastfeeding should be carefully assessed if the infant
    a. continues to lose weight on days 5 and 6.
    b. loses up to 7 percent of his birth weight.
    c. does not regain birth weight until day 14.
    d. has a birth weight greater than 9 lb.

12. It is common for thriving infants to be wakeful and feed frequently (in "clusters") in the
    a. morning, after dawn.
    b. early afternoon.

    c. late afternoon or early evening.

    d. middle of the night.

13. When an infant feeds much more frequently than usual for a few days, breastmilk is synthesized

    a. more rapidly than the norm, to keep up with the rate of withdrawal.

    b. less rapidly than the norm, because frequent feeds compensate so that the baby maintains his normal intake.

    c. less rapidly than the norm, thus producing a high fat concentration

    d. at about the same rate as usual.

14. Which practice has the potential to increase a mother's milk supply?

    a. scheduled feedings

    b. expression of residual milk after feedings

    c. use of supplemental feedings

    d. infant use of pacifiers

15. As compared with larger-breasted women, breastfeeding mothers who have small breasts

    a. have little subcutaneous fat, but have about the same milk storage capacity.

    b. will likely feed their infants more frequently per 24 hours.

    c. will likely feed their infants less frequently per 24 hours.

    d. will likely feed their infants about the same number of times per 24 hours.

16. Prompt lactogenesis II is promoted by

    a. intact anterior pituitary.

    b. insulin-dependent diabetes.

    c. cesarean delivery.

    d. obesity.

17. A woman who synthesizes sufficient breastmilk for her singleton infant can do so even if she also experiences

    a. retained placenta.

    b. lack of pituitary prolactin.

    c. lack of pituitary oxytocin.

    d. severed nerves that innervate the nipple.

18. A baby who consistently chokes during milk letdown is most likely responding to

    a. delayed maternal letdown reflex.

    b. feeding in an upright position.

    c. difficulty in coordinating swallowing and breathing.

    d. small infant oral space.

19. A mother with a superabundant milk supply can increase her infant's comfort during feeding by
    a. offering both breasts at each feeding.
    b. positioning the baby's head below the breast.
    c. feeding at as long intervals as the baby will tolerate.
    d. removing the baby during her initial milk letdown.

20. Nipple pain is more likely to be experienced by women who
    a. did not prepare their nipples prenatally.
    b. have fair skin or hair.
    c. are primiparous.
    d. feed for long periods of time.

21. Short breastfeeding bouts in the early postpartum lead to
    a. transfer of larger volumes of milk to the infant.
    b. transfer of smaller volumes of hindmilk to the infant.
    c. lesser likelihood of damaged nipple skin.
    d. early-onset nipple soreness.

22. When it is positioned in the baby's mouth for effective breastfeeding, the nipple
    a. flattens between the tongue and roof of the mouth but stretches very little.
    b. doubles its length and the tip becomes wedge shaped.
    c. elongates so that the nipple pores are near the edge of the soft palate.
    d. lengthens and the end of the nipple rests on the tongue about midway between gums and pharynx.

23. During suck-swallow-breathe episodes, milk flows into the baby's mouth fastest during the
    a. upward movement of the baby's jaw.
    b. downward movement of the baby's jaw.
    c. pause between suck-swallow-breathe episodes.
    d. breathing interval.

24. A breastfeeding infant normally makes which sound during feeding?
    a. clicking   c. slurping
    b. aaaaah   d. none

25. A useful way to reduce nipple pain or damage during early breastfeeding is to
    a. limit the length of breastfeeds.
    b. limit the duration of breastfeeds.
    c. let the baby suck on a pacifier instead of the breast.
    d. make sure that the baby takes a big mouthful of breast.

26. With respect to breastfeeding, the term "storage capacity" refers to the
    a. amount of milk that a baby's stomach can hold at a given feeding.
    b. amount of extracellular fluid stored in a well-hydrated infant.
    c. minimum amount of extracellular fluid stored in an infant, below which an infant is considered dehydrated.
    d. amount of milk that a breast can comfortably store.

27. Breasts will begin to involute if
    a. only about 80% of the milk in the breast is removed consistently.
    b. components in the milk promote proliferation of lactocytes.
    c. distension of the lumen of the milk alveoli disrupts the lactocytes.
    d. they have excess milk storage capacity.

28. Milk stasis can lead to
    a. cysts in milk ducts.
    b. pressure straightening of distal milk-collecting ducts.
    c. infectious mastitis.
    d. peau d'orange texture in breast skin.

29. After full breastmilk feedings are established, the neonate's stools become
    a. black and firm.
    b. greenish and sticky.
    c. greenish and firm.
    d. yellow and very soft.

30. The distressing infant crying that signals infant colic may be
    a. reduced by increased carrying.
    b. increased by carrying prone on a parent's forearm.
    c. reduced by unwrapping the infant.
    d. increased by small amounts of oral sucrose.

31. By 2 weeks of age, what fecal flora predominate in breastfed infants?
    a. bifidobacteria and lactobacili
    b. lactobacili and enterococci
    c. enterococci and coliforms
    d. coliforms and bifidobacteria

32. During the first 6 months or so of breastfeeding, the whey:casein ratio of human milk
    a. stays constant at 80:20.
    b. increases from about 60:40 to about 90:10.
    c. decreases from about 90:10 to about 60:40.
    d. moderates other changes in breastmilk composition so that the consistency of stools does not change.

33. Physiological jaundice
    a. affects only a small percentage of newborns.
    b. becomes apparent in the first 24 hours of life.
    c. peaks shortly after breastmilk comes in.
    d. requires intervention in the majority of affected infants.

34. In a breastfeeding week-old infant, exaggerated physiological jaundice is associated with
    a. more than 8 feedings per 24 hours.
    b. a need for water supplements.
    c. audible swallowing sounds during feedings.
    d. a baby who quickly falls asleep at the breast.

35. Young infants who, for unexplained reasons, suddenly refuse to take the breast may be induced to return to breastfeeding by
    a. withholding the breast and using alternate feeding methods until the infant signals readiness to breastfeed.
    b. withholding all feedings until the infant is hungry enough to breastfeed.
    c. offering the breast when the infant is drowsy.
    d. offering the breast in a way that minimizes skin-to-skin contact.

36. A common first response to a crying baby is to offer the breast, because
    a. the baby cannot cry and feed simultaneously.
    b. suckling at the breast is analgesic.
    c. the mother's breast is slightly cooler than her body, preventing overheating of a stimulated baby.
    d. the nutritive content of breastmilk replaces the large amount of energy expended in crying.

37. The allergen most commonly ingested by infants is
    a. cow milk.   c. chicken.
    b. soy-based formula.   d. eggs.

38. Breastfeeding infants who develop colic symptoms in response to certain foods in their mother's diet are, later in life,
    a. protected against allergic reactions to those foods.
    b. likely to show allergic reactions to those foods.
    c. at no increased or decreased risk of showing allergic reactions to those foods.
    d. at greater risk of obesity.

39. Lactation specialists are increasingly likely to work with mothers of twins or triplets (or higher-order births) because
    a. mothers of multiples initiate breastfeeding at about the same rate as mothers of singletons.
    b. those infants are more apt to be released from the hospital before they breastfeed well.

    c. environmental factors currently make it more likely that a women will produce two or more mature ova when she ovulates.

    d. twins or triplets are more apt to be born to younger mothers, who are still developing their breast tissue.

40. Continuing to breastfeed an 18-month-old infant during a subsequent pregnancy should be discouraged because

    a. of the hazard of miscarriage, even in a healthy pregnancy.

    b. it places the older infant at a nutritional risk.

    c. it places a debilitating energy demand on the mother.

    d. of the risk of miscarriage, if the mother is at risk for preterm labor.

41. Mothers who continue to breastfeed an older child during a subsequent pregnancy commonly experience

    a. an increase in energy.

    b. diminished milk supply.

    c. an increase in nipple comfort.

    d. diminished nursings by the child.

42. In order to assure herself that her 8-week-old breastfeeding infant is taking enough breastmilk, a mother can look for

    a. breasts that remain full after a feeding.

    b. 4 to 6 effective breastfeeds per 24 hours.

    c. 1 or 2 soft stools per 24 hours.

    d. at least 6 heavy wet diapers per 24 hours.

43. By about 6 weeks postpartum, the mother's milk supply adjusts relative to the baby so that

    a. the baby must increase her number of feedings per day to consume adequate volumes of milk.

    b. the fat content of the milk is higher, and the baby thrives on fewer feeds per day.

    c. the breast retains about 25% of its milk to allow for occasional larger feedings.

    d. the breast retains about 25% of its milk, indicating the need to begin supplemental feeds.

44. Nipple pain in the first few days postpartum is BEST treated by

    a. topical antibiotics to heal any micro-abrasions in the nipple skin.

    b. breast shells to keep clothing from irritating the nipple skin.

    c. correcting the position of the infant's mouth on the breast.

    d. rubbing breastmilk into the nipple skin.

45. Infant behavior at the breast that suggests milk oversupply may also be caused by a

    a. baby who nurses too vigorously.

    b. maternal diet too rich in fat.

    c. baby who does not coordinate suckling and breathing well.

    d. mother whose body is compensating for painful nipples.

46. Crying in a young infant
    a. is a late sign of hunger.
    b. is an early sign of hunger.
    c. promotes general infant vigor.
    d. promotes good oxygenation.

Discussion Questions

1. What is the normal pattern of weight change in the first 2 weeks of an infant's life? What is the latest day that a baby should begin regaining weight? What percent weight loss is a marker for further evaluation? What is the latest day by which birth weight should be regained?

2. What are cluster feedings? Are they cause for alarm? How should they best be handled?

3. How are severe postpartum hemorrhage and later breastfeeding difficulties related?

4. Contrast typical stooling patterns in an exclusively breastfed baby and a baby exclusively fed manufactured milks at the following time points:
    a. day 2   d. 1 month
    b. day 5   e. 3 months
    c. 2 weeks

5. How do you respond to a mother who thinks she doesn't have enough milk for her 3-month-old baby? The baby is at the 75th percentile for height and the 50th percentile for weight.
    a. What might the baby be doing to make the mother draw this conclusion? Discuss at least five factors.
    b. What might the mother be doing or feeling to make her draw this conclusion? Discuss at least five factors.

6. How do you decide whether "sore nipples" are transient and normal or are prolonged and abnormal? What might cause each case? What would you suggest to resolve each one?

7. Why do babies sometimes refuse the breast? Suggest at least three reasons; consider infants at various ages. What would you suggest to return the baby to the breast?

8. What is overactive letdown reflex? Is it a problem? Why or why not? How can the mother cope with it?

9. What information about breastfeeding should be discussed as part of a hospital discharge plan for a postpartum woman?

10. What community services or organizations can you recommend to a new breastfeeding mother who is now at home?

BREAST-RELATED PROBLEMS

Atypical physical characteristics of the breast, either temporary or permanent, can render breastfeeding more difficult. This chapter describes how to recognize, manage, or compensate for atypical presentations of the exterior skin and the interior tissues of the breast that impinge upon breastfeeding. Questions in this chapter will help you to assess your understanding of this body of information and how it applies to professional practice.

Chapter Outline

Multiple-Choice Questions

1. Retractile inverted nipples

    a. are so firmly inverted that they cannot be pulled out.

    b. may be caused to evert more easily by the changes of pregnancy.

    c. make it very difficult for a baby to draw the nipple into her mouth.

    d. are inverted when at rest and after manipulation.

2. If the mother has an inverted nipple

    a. the nursing baby usually suckles and obtains milk.

    b. the breast does not function well; thus, lactation should not be attempted.

    c. the breast produces milk, but the nipple does not function sufficiently to sustain the infant.

    d. breastfeeding proceeds more easily with the first baby than with later ones, for whom the inversion typically becomes more severe.

3. Exceptionally long maternal nipples

    a. require that the nursing infant work harder to obtain milk because the ducts are narrow in the nipple.

    b. may prevent large neonates from grasping the areola.

    c. may trigger a gag reflex in susceptible infants.

    d. are more common in women of Mediterranean descent.

4. Plugged ducts are commonly associated with

    a. a marginally adequate milk supply that results in frequent breastfeeds and thus many letdowns.

    b. localized tenderness in one area of the breast and generalized fever.

    c. a palpable lump in the breast and a generalized fever.

    d. a baby who does not regularly take most of the milk in the breast.

5. A plugged duct may be resolved by
   a. firmly massaging the tender area after breastfeeds.
   b. positioning the baby at the breast so that his nose points toward the tender region.
   c. breastfeeding less frequently to increase milk pressure behind the plug.
   d. breastfeeding less frequently to avoid stimulating multiple letdowns that cause milk to back up in a duct.

6. A mother who has nipple rashes is apt to benefit MOST from
   a. about 15 minutes per day of sunlight on her nipples.
   b. wearing shirts and brassieres made of fabrics that "breathe."
   c. use, after a feed, of a hair dryer set on "warm" to dry unrinsed nipples.
   d. rinsing the nipples with warm water after each feeding.

7. Mothers are most likely to rate which of the following factors as the most important precursor of mastitis?
   a. plugged duct
   b. cracked nipple
   c. fatigue
   d. milk stasis

8. Mastitis is usually characterized by
   a. a fever, rapid pulse, and inversion of the nipple on the affected side.
   b. bilateral tenderness and streaks moving from each nipple up the breast.
   c. a feeling that the breast is colder than usual.
   d. localized breast tenderness, usually unilateral; fatigue; and muscular aching.

9. Temporarily stopping breastfeeding by a mother who has mastitis will
   a. remove a definite risk to the baby from ingesting infected milk.
   b. allow any medications that the mother uses to remain in the breast longer and will hasten her recovery.
   c. delay the mother's recovery, unless she pumps as much milk as the baby usually takes.
   d. allow the breast to overfill, thus diluting the infected fluids in the breast, which will benefit the infant.

10. During an active breast infection, the composition of breastmilk changes such that
    a. anti-inflammatory agents, sodium, and chloride all decrease.
    b. anti-inflammatory agents and sodium increase, but chloride decreases.
    c. anti-inflammatory agents and chloride decrease, but sodium increases.
    d. anti-inflammatory agents, sodium, and chloride all increase.

11. A breast abscess
    a. is the outcome of approximately 90 percent of cases of mastitis.
    b. spells the end of breastfeeding on the affected side if surgical drainage is required.

    c. generally is associated with streptococcal bacteria in the breast.

    d. may require incision and drainage, after which breastfeeding can be resumed.

12. Yeast infections (candidiasis) may present with

    a. generalized fever, deep pink nipples, and severe pain during and immediately after breastfeeding.

    b. deep pink inflammation of the nipples, severe pain during and immediately after breastfeeding, and bright red pustular diaper rash in the infant.

    c. severe pain during and immediately after breastfeeding, bright red pustular diaper rash in the infant, and generalized fever.

    d. bright red pustular diaper rash in the infant, generalized fever, and deep pink inflammation of the nipples.

13. In order to eliminate a woman's recurrent yeast infection, which of the following should be treated?

    a. the woman only

    b. the woman and her sexual partner

    c. the woman, her sexual partner, and the baby

    d. the woman, her sexual partner, the baby, and items that regularly go into the baby's mouth

14. A woman who had surgery that changed her breast size generally will have the BEST chance of fully breastfeeding if

    a. only the fourth intercostal nerves were severed.

    b. only blood vessels to the areola complex, rather than to lactocytes, were severed.

    c. the breast was augmented rather than reduced.

    d. the breast was reduced rather than augmented.

15. After breast reduction surgery, a woman has the LEAST chance of producing adequate breastmilk if

    a. the free-nipple technique of breast reconstruction was used.

    b. only a small amount of gland was removed.

    c. the sixth intercostal nerve was severed.

    d. the seventh intercostal nerve was severed.

16. Breast reduction or augmentation surgery will result in

    a. no effect on milk transfer if the mother has periareolar surgery.

    b. low likelihood of sufficient milk transfer following periareolar surgery.

    c. no effect on milk transfer if the mother has previously breastfed.

    d. no effect on milk transfer unless the mother gives birth prematurely.

17. Milk ducts severed during breast reduction surgery usually

    a. do not hinder breastfeeding, because the severed ends tend to reattach.

    b. do not hinder breastfeeding, because the severed end with milk in it attaches to an intact and flowing duct.

    c. do hinder breastfeeding, because the severed ducts spill milk into breast tissue, which is more likely to develop mastitis.

    d. do hinder breastfeeding, because pressure atrophy of glands feeding into that duct may reduce milk supply.

18. A red tinge to breastmilk

    a. usually means that the mother has eaten red foods in the previous 18 to 24 hours.

    b. is caused by thinner milk ducts in multiparous women, which allow blood to leak into the ducts.

    c. is most common in primiparous women during early days of breastfeeding.

    d. from whatever cause means that the baby should be weaned to avoid ingesting blood.

19. Recommend that a lactating woman be examined by her health-care provider if she notices

    a. a persistent difference in breast size.

    b. a breast lump that does not change during 3 days of normal breastfeeding.

    c. cracked nipples that leak blood into her breastmilk.

    d. bouts of mastitis that move to different locations in the breasts.

20. Studies show that having breastfed an infant and subsequent development of breast cancer

    a. are directly related in postmenopausal women.

    b. are inversely related in premenopausal women.

    c. are directly related in both premenopausal and postmenopausal women.

    d. bear no statistical relationship to each other in either premenopausal or postmenopausal women.

21. A diagnostic sign of a developing cancerous lump in the breast is

    a. breast tenderness.

    b. enlargement of breast alveoli.

    c. increased breast-tissue density.

    d. peau d'orange skin texture.

22. Infants who are inadvertently fed on a cancerous breast

    a. rarely gain weight at the normal rate.

    b. rarely increase in length at the normal rate.

    c. may reject a cancerous breast without apparent reason.

    d. tend to prefer to nurse on a cancerous breast.

23. Women currently being treated by chemotherapy for any cancer should be encouraged to

    a. breastfeed because the drugs do not pass from her system into breastmilk.

    b. not breastfeed because common chemotherapy drugs pass into milk and will harm the infant.

    c. breastfeed because the chemotherapy drugs are destroyed in the infant's stomach.

    d. not breastfeed because the mother's system still contains cancer-causing agents.

24. Women who have been treated for unilateral breast cancer
    a. should not breastfeed a later child at all to avoid passing along cancer-causing agents in the milk.
    b. should not feed from the affected breast to avoid passing along cancer-causing agents in the milk.
    c. are less likely to produce a full milk supply from the treated breast.
    d. are rarely able to produce milk with sufficient fats for the baby to grow.

25. After a breastfeeding mother has had surgery on a breast, such as removal of a lump or drainage of an abscess, she should
    a. resume breastfeeding on both breasts as soon as she can do so comfortably.
    b. resume breastfeeding only if the baby also has some other form of nourishment.
    c. pump her milk until all drainage from the incision site has ended.
    d. resume breastfeeding only on the intact breast.

Discussion Questions

1. Describe at least five ways to treat a plugged duct.

2. What is a fibrocystic breast condition? Is it a contraindication to breastfeeding? Provide the rationale for your response.

3. What is an intraductal papilloma? How is it identified, and what is its effect on lactation?

4. What factors seem to predispose women to develop mastitis? Discuss at least four factors and emphasize interactions among factors.

5. What is a nipple blister? How is it recognized? How should it be treated?

6. What is candidiasis? How is it identified? In what regions of the body can candidiasis (thrush) lodge? In what members of the family can it be found?

7. What is a common (although by no means universal) cause of lumps in the lactating breast? What procedures are use to determine if breast lumps are cancerous or benign? Does breastfeeding need to be interrupted or terminated if such a procedure is to be performed?

8. Do breastfeeding women (or women who have breastfed) get breast cancer? Is it harmful for an infant to breastfeed if his mother has (or has had) breast cancer? Explain the rationale for your response.

Low Intake in the Breastfed Infant: Maternal and Infant Considerations

"Low intake" here refers not to some fixed volume of breastmilk, but to the adequacy of intake as compared with the infant's needs. A baby whose weight gain is inadequate must be assessed in relation to his mother: Either may be the independent cause of poor infant weight gain. Even so, their intimate interaction produces responses in each other that may exacerbate the infant's condition. Questions in this chapter will help you to assess your understanding of how to evaluate and manage the breastfeeding dyad when the infant's intake is inadequate.

Chapter Outline

Factors that Influence Maternal Milk Production

Normal Milk Intake and Rate of Gain

US Growth Curves

    Current growth curves still underrepresent breastfeeding

Low Intake and Low Milk Supply: Definitions and Incidence of Occurrence

    Confusing terminology and nonstandardized research

    The infant's presentation

    The mother's presentation

Abnormal Patterns of Growth: The Baby Who Appears Healthy

    Inadequate weight gain in the first month

    The near-term infant

    Oral-motor dysfunction (ineffective suckling)

Multiple-Choice Questions

1. On the basis of currently available (2004) growth charts, between 4 and 12 months of age, fully breastfed infants generally weigh
   a. about the same as formula-fed infants.
   b. more than formula-fed infants.
   c. less than formula-fed infants.
   d. less than formula-fed infants until solids are well established.

2. At 1 month of age, both breastfed and formula-fed infants gain about _____ per day.
   a. 1/2 ounce
   b. 1 ounce
   c. 2 ounces
   d. 3 ounces

3. Maternal nutritional status bears
   a. a strong direct relationship with milk volume.
   b. a strong direct relationship with fat content.
   c. an inverse relationship with milk volume.
   d. little correlation with milk volume.

4. Exclusively breastfed infants between 1 and 9 months of age anywhere in the world consume, on average, about what volume of milk per day?
   a. 15 ounces (450 ml)
   b. 25 ounces (755 ml)
   c. 35 ounces (1050 ml)
   d. 55 ounces (1650 ml)

5. As compared with infants fed manufactured milks, during the first 3 months fully breastfed infants
   a. consume less milk but grow at the same rates.
   b. consume about the same amount of milk and grow at the same rates.
   c. consume more milk and grow at faster rates.
   d. consume less milk and grow at slower rates.

6. Which of the following growth parameters is most likely to suggest early failure to thrive?
   a. infant weight
   b. infant head circumference
   c. length/height
   d. chest circumference

7. A healthy neonate who weighed 7 lb at birth and weighs 6 lb 4 oz at 8 days of age
   a. is doing OK, considering that the mother's milk has been "in" for only 4 days.
   b. is unlikely to be jaundiced.
   c. should be evaluated, along with her mother, for possible breastfeeding problems.
   d. will have several large stools per day.

8. Weight loss above _____ of birth weight and failure to regain birth weight by _____ postpartum both require thorough assessment and intervention.

   a. 5 percent, 7 days
   c. 5 percent, 14 days
   b. 10 percent, 8 days
   d. 10 percent, 14 days

9. During the first 4 weeks, the root cause of poor weight gain in a breastfeeding infant is

   a. more likely to be feeding problems than underlying infant illness.

   b. more likely to be underlying infant illness than feeding problems.

   c. equally likely to be feeding problems and underlying illness.

   d. more likely to be maternal indifference than underlying infant illness.

10. American Academy of Pediatrics guidelines state that a breastfeeding infant released from the hospital before 48 hours of age must be seen by a health professional on postpartum day

    a. 3, 4, or 5
    c. 10
    b. 7
    d. 14

11. A chief complaint about the US standard growth charts used before year 2000 is that they were based on

    a. less reliable statistical methods.

    b. a sample of infants most of whom were fed manufactured milks.

    c. a sample of infants from a variety of ethnic backgrounds.

    d. a sample of infants from a variety of locations in the United States.

12. As compared with a healthy full-term newborn, a healthy infant who is born at 36 weeks gestation, 2800 g birth weight, and without medical complications is

    a. less likely to experience excessive weight loss or jaundice.

    b. about as likely to experience excessive weight loss or jaundice.

    c. very slightly more likely to experience excessive weight loss or jaundice.

    d. significantly more likely to experience excessive weight loss or jaundice.

13. As the rate of milk flow _____, the rate of infant suckling _____.

    a. increases, increases

    b. increases, decreases

    c. decreases, decreases

    d. decreases, stays the same

14. A baby with low overall muscle tone may also exhibit

    a. jaw clenching.

    b. biting.

    c. weak suction.

    d. compression of the nipple against his palate.

15. In nearly all cases, milk production is related more to
    a. effective breastfeeding by the baby than to maternal ability to make milk.
    b. maternal ability to make milk than to effective breastfeeding by the baby.
    c. maternal nutritional status than to size of the baby at birth.
    d. size of the baby at birth than to maternal nutritional status.

16. A breastfeeding baby may be chronically unsettled for all of the following reasons EXCEPT
    a. allergy to a food in the mother's diet.
    b. maternal milk supply far exceeding the infant's need.
    c. gastroesophegeal reflux.
    d. sensitivity to breastmilk lipids.

17. Maternal breastmilk oversupply may be suggested by a baby who has
    a. long quiet, contented intervals.
    b. frequent watery stools.
    c. a growth rate at the 90th percentile or higher.
    d. difficulty initially latching onto the nipple at each feed.

18. An infant who has a short, tight frenulum may
    a. have difficulty raising the back of the tongue to meet the back of the hard palate.
    b. have a point at the tip of the tongue.
    c. be unable to move the tongue forward to cover the gum ridge.
    d. create an exceptionally tight seal around the breast.

19. Mothers in whom lactogenesis II is delayed beyond the third day postpartum may experience a chronic low milk supply because
    a. the delay in lactogenesis II is caused by the same hormonal factors that cause milk to be synthesized at a slower-than-usual rate during full lactation.
    b. infants of these mothers are more likely to receive supplements by feeding bottle before their mothers' milk comes in.
    c. delayed lactogenesis is more common in women who have small breasts.
    d. their infants are typically large and have ample body stores and thus little early urge to suckle.

20. After documentation of inverted nipples in a pregnant woman, the lactation consultant should
    a. recommend methods for everting the nipple, because treatment is necessary to ensure that the infant will be able to latch on properly.
    b. not recommend methods for everting the nipple, because the treatments never succeed.
    c. tell the woman not to worry because inverted nipples rarely cause breastfeeding problems.
    d. be available for supportive care during the early days of breastfeeding.

21. Use of a thin silicone nipple shield is MOST likely to

    a. increase milk transfer by enabling an infant to more easily grasp the nipple.

    b. increase the discomfort of a mother with very sore nipples.

    c. decrease milk transfer by triggering an infant's gag reflex.

    d. eliminate the need to pump the breasts.

22. A mother who has a very low milk supply, but whose newborn is healthy and nursing appropriately, may have

    a. a fragment of placenta retained in the uterus.

    b. high thyroid concentrations in the blood.

    c. low prolactin concentrations in the blood.

    d. just begun taking progesterone-only contraceptives.

23. Breast augmentation surgery is associated with difficulty in sustaining an infant at the breast, in part because this surgery may be a marker for

    a. lack of real interest in breastfeeding.

    b. breasts that lack milk-producing glandular tissue.

    c. true inverted nipples–nipples that cannot be pulled out and thus are difficult to latch on to.

    d. low levels of prolactin.

24. An amount of glandular tissue in the breast insufficient to support a nursing infant is a problem

    a. for at least 5 percent of women in the developed world.

    b. that explains nearly all infant failure to thrive.

    c. that is quite rare.

    d. that is usually secondary to chest trauma.

25. Inadequate nutrition in the pregnant mother is associated with lower than normal milk volumes because

    a. the mother did not accumulate adequate calorie stores.

    b. the mother did not accumulate adequate fluid stores.

    c. the baby is small for gestational age and takes less milk.

    d. the baby is appropriate for gestational age but relatively inactive.

Discussion Questions

1. What is tongue-tie? How do you identify it? If it is not treated, what are the consequences for breastfeeding? How is tongue-tie corrected?

2. What are the common consequences to breastfeeding of the following situations?

    a. pregnancy superimposed on lactation

    b. contraceptive pills begun early in lactation

    c. smoking

    d. hypothyroidism

e. hyperthyroidism

f. alcohol ingestion

What mechanism of action produces those consequences?

3. What factors predispose a postpartum woman to delayed lactogenesis II? Describe four maternal factors and two infant factors.

4. What is the importance of listening for infant swallowing when one is evaluating a slow-gaining infant?

5. How might disorganized suckling in a newborn affect the establishment of breastfeeding? What might have caused this disorganization? What practices will help to establish breastfeeding in the face of a disorganized suck?

6. What is the relationship between poor infant weight gain and low maternal milk volumes? Describe conditions that might make the mother the independent variable; then describe conditions that might make the infant the independent variable.

7. What are the two most obvious indicators of inadequate breastmilk intake by an infant?

8. What is the difference between a "slow gaining" baby and a "failure-to-thrive" baby? How do standard growth curves play into this diagnosis? Are standard growth curves adequate for assessing breastfed infants?

9. During their first year, are breastfed babies underfed or are babies fed manufactured milks overfed? What is the rationale for your response? Do breastfed infants "falter" in growth around 3 or 4 months of age?

10. How does a mother's nutritional status during lactation affect her milk volumes?

11. How would you distinguish between a satiated baby, a sleepy baby, and a baby who is suffering from failure to thrive, when all have their eyes closed while at the breast?

12. Describe at least four infant health conditions that can result in failure to thrive. How can the condition be recognized? How can breastfeeding still be maintained?

13. What is the role of nighttime feedings in promoting adequate infant weight gain? What is the physiological basis for this role?

JAUNDICE AND THE BREASTFED BABY

Jaundice is the great conundrum of early breastfeeding: How can the perfect infant food sometimes lead to a possibly life-threatening illness in the neonate? The lactation consultant should be able to distinguish between common physiologic jaundice, "nonbreastfeeding" jaundice, and pathologic jaundice and understand how each is managed. Questions in this chapter will help you to assess your understanding of this body of information and how it applies to professional practice.

Chapter Outline

Neonatal Jaundice

Assessment of Jaundice

Postnatal Patterns of Jaundice

Breastmilk Jaundice

Breast-Nonfeeding Jaundice

Bilirubin Encephalopathy

Evaluation of Jaundice

   Diagnostic assessment

Management of Jaundice

Key Concepts

Internet Resources

References

Multiple-Choice Questions

1. One feature of jaundice is

   a. a deep reddish tinge to the skin.

   b. increased excretion of bilirubin.

    c. deposition of biliverdin in tissues.

    d. increased hemoglobin breakdown.

2. Physiologic jaundice

    a. occurs in more than half of full-term, healthy infants.

    b. is more common in formula-fed than in breastfed infants.

    c. is experienced by only about 25 percent of all newborns.

    d. persists beyond 7 days of birth for almost all full-term infants.

3. "Starvation-induced" jaundice in a breastfed infant is

    a. uncommon but possible on day one of life.

    b. more likely if rate of milk transfer is low.

    c. common in infants given frequent milk feedings.

    d. is an early manifestation of cow-milk allergy.

4. Clinical jaundice in the 5-day-old term neonate means that

    a. more bilirubin is produced than is eliminated.

    b. more bilirubin is eliminated than produced.

    c. almost equal amounts of bilirubin are produced and eliminated.

    d. elimination of bilirubin production has stopped.

5. Three-day-old healthy newborns of which of the following groups are likely to have the highest average bilirubin levels?

    a. Asian

    b. Hispanic

    c. Caucasian

    d. Sub-Saharan African

6. Which of the following factors is LEAST likely to promote jaundice?

    a. induction of labor

    b. mother with diabetes

    c. cephalhematoma

    d. appropriate for gestational age term birth

7. Physiologic jaundice

    a. is a condition commonly seen in healthy term newborns.

    b. is apparent first in yellow-tinged nailbeds.

    c. results from the deposition of a yellow molecule (biliverdin) in tissue.

    d. commonly becomes apparent in the first 24 hours of life.

8. Breastmilk jaundice typically

    a. occurs only in compromised breastfed infants.

    b. manifests at about 14 days of age.

    c. is a sign of underlying medical problems.

    d. is a longer-lasting version of physiologic jaundice.

9. "Breast-nonfeeding jaundice" describes a condition in neonates who

    a. receive no feedings of breast fluids and are fed only artificial milks.

    b. pass abundant stools that reduce the intestinal lining's ability to extract nutrients from the milk.

    c. ingest low breastmilk volumes and retain fecal material.

    d. are breastfeeding and simply have physiologic jaundice.

10. As compared with thriving formula-fed neonates at day seven of life, thriving breastfed neonates fed on demand have a

    a. similar rate of elevated bilirubin and similar average weight loss.

    b. lower rate of elevated bilirubin but greater average weight loss.

    c. higher rate of elevated bilirubin but lower average weight loss.

    d. higher rate of elevated bilirubin and similar average weight loss.

11. Infants who develop "breast-nonfeeding" jaundice in the first several days of life are

    a. thereby protected from excessively high concentrations of bilirubin if they go on to develop breast-milk jaundice.

    b. at average risk of developing excessively high concentrations of bilirubin if they go on to develop breastmilk jaundice.

    c. at higher risk of developing excessively high concentrations of bilirubin if they go on to develop breastmilk jaundice.

    d. extremely unlikely to develop a different type of jaundice once the volume of ingested milk increases.

12. As compared with adults, healthy newborns typically have higher serum bilirubin concentrations in part because

    a. the newborn liver and intestines promote recirculation of bilirubin.

    b. newborns have a smaller red blood cell mass at birth.

    c. the red blood cells of newborns have longer life spans.

    d. the newborn liver binds bilirubin more rapidly.

13. Judging an infant's degree of jaundice by visual inspection

    a. relies on progressive yellowing of skin from the head to the lower extremities as bilirubin concentration increases.

    b. is a reliable way to estimate unconjugated serum bilirubin.

    c. is a reliable way to estimate conjugated serum bilirubin.

    d. is reliable regardless of an infant's ethnicity.

14. Bilirubin levels commonly peak

    a. around day five in healthy Caucasian infants.

    b. at lower levels in Asian newborns than in Caucasian newborns.

    c. earlier in preterm newborns than in full-term newborns.

    d. earlier in Caucasian newborns than in Asian newborns.

15. Jaundice in an infant less than 24 hours old usually can be attributed to

    a. breastmilk jaundice.

    b. "breast-nonfeeding" jaundice.

    c. an underlying medical problem.

    d. side effects of maternal epidural anesthesia.

16. Kernicterus–bilirubin staining of brain tissue–is

    a. no longer a public health issue since the advent of phototherapy.

    b. less likely in breastfeeding infants because of protective factors in breastmilk.

    c. a greater risk for infants who experience early "breast-nonfeeding" jaundice.

    d. a condition that the baby will eventually grow out of.

17. The form of bilirubin that stains brain tissues is

    a. conjugated (bound) bilirubin.

    b. unconjugated and unbound bilirubin.

    c. a bilirubin stereoisomer.

    d. a biliverdin molecule.

18. Elevated bilirubin levels may be promoted by

    a. breakdown of smaller numbers of red blood cells than the liver can process.

    b. infrequent stooling.

    c. feedings of manufactured milks.

    d. higher than usual levels of bilirubin bound to plasma proteins.

19. Phototherapy is used to treat some jaundiced infants because the wavelengths of light used in phototherapy

    a. stimulate infant appetite, which promotes stooling.

    b. promote peristalsis and thus stooling.

    c. alter the bilirubin molecule to one that is more easily excreted.

    d. reduce the rate at which red blood cells break down.

20. Breastfed infants receiving phototherapy should

    a. continue to be breastfed.

    b. be weaned to formula.

    c. be switched to formula for the duration of phototherapy.

    d. be fed intravenously as a matter of course.

Discussion Questions

1. How will answers to each of the following questions help you evaluate an infant's risk of early-onset infant jaundice?

   a. How many times is the infant put to breast in 24 hours?

   b. How effectively is the baby suckling?

   c. What is the baby's stooling pattern?

   d. Besides breastmilk, what other fluids is the baby being given?

   e. When is the baby being breastfed during any 24-hour period?

   f. Are the mother's nipples comfortable?

2. How does ethnicity affect normal serum bilirubin levels in newborn infants? How do these differences affect the care given those infants?

3. Should breastfeeding be interrupted for a day or two to reduce serum bilirubin levels in infants being treated under bili-lights? Is it ever reasonable to briefly interrupt use of bilirubin lights in order to feed or comfort the treated infant?

4. How can "normal" early jaundice, pathological jaundice, and breastmilk jaundice be distinguished?

5. Why are infants fed manufactured milks less likely to receive a diagnosis of jaundice in the first few days of life? Is this fact sufficient justfication for feeding artificial milks during this interval?

6. How does each of the following characteristics of infants influence the likelihood that a baby will receive a diagnosis of early-onset jaundice?

   a. racial or ethnic group

   b. birth weight

   c. stool patterns

   d. weight loss

7. How might hospital routines that determine the following influence the likelihood of severe hyperbilirubinemia developing in an infant?

   a. use of analgesia or anesthesia

   b. type of infant feeding

   c. frequency of feeding

   d. supplemental milk feedings

   e. supplemental water feedings

Breast Pumps and Other Technologies

Babies are the best breastmilk extractor, but babies are not always available when milk needs to be removed. Specialized pumps are increasingly used to obtain milk and sustain the milk-producing capacity of the breast in both short-term and long-term situations. Lactation consultants should understand the principles upon which various types of pumps work and how to fit a pump to the mother for optimal performance. Questions in this chapter will help you to assess your understanding of this body of information and how it applies to professional practice.

Chapter Outline

Multiple-Choice Questions

1. For optimal response to a breast pump, the milk-ejection reflex should be elicited
   a. before the mother begins pumping her breasts.
   b. at the time the mother begins pumping her breast.
   c. after the mother has been pumping her breast at least 2 minutes.
   d. whenever milk begins to flow during the pumping session.

2. A lactation consultant who recommends that a mother use nipple shields should also
   a. ask the mother to sign a consent form identifying the risks of using the device.
   b. suggest that nipple shields should be used until the baby weans.
   c. note that only neurologically impaired babies benefit from their use.
   d. note that the shield will alter the baby's suck, preventing later attachment to the breast.

3. A mother is most likely to pump the most milk in a single pumping session
   a. in the evening.
   b. shortly after awakening in the morning.
   c. shortly after the baby has breastfed.
   d. whenever she has waited at least 3 hours since the last pumping session.

4. Volumes of milk pumped are likely to
   a. be independent of the mother's emotional state.
   b. increase a little as the mother's degree of emotional stress increases.
   c. decrease markedly as the mother's degree of emotional stress increases.
   d. decrease with increasing stress, but only very slightly.

5. In order for a baby to use a feeding-tube device effectively, the baby
   a. should be able to latch onto the breast and suckle.
   b. need not be able to latch but should be able to protect his airway.
   c. should not be jaundiced.
   d. should be at least 39 weeks' gestational age.

6. A technique that promotes increased volumes of pumped milk is
   a. exercising vigorously shortly before pumping.
   b. pumping at least 5 minutes after the last drop of milk has been expressed, to ensure that all possible milk has been taken.
   c. applying cool compresses to the breasts to increase tissue contraction.
   d. massaging the breasts during pumping to increase intramammary pressure.

7. The principal mechanism by which pumps cause milk to flow from the breast is by
   a. suction, like sucking on a straw.
   b. mechanical kneading of the breast that squeezes milk out.
   c. mimicking the sensations produced by a baby at the breast.
   d. creating a pressure gradient down which milk flows.

8. As compared with a baby at the breast, a breast pump usually stimulates the milk ejection reflex
   a. in about the same length of time.
   b. in a considerably longer time.
   c. in a shorter period of time.
   d. in less and less time as pumping continues.

9. Pumping the breasts after milk stops flowing or dripping
   a. will promote further letdowns at that pumping episode.
   b. will markedly increase future milk supply.
   c. is likely to damage breast tissue.
   d. ensures that nipples will remain everted.

10. If she is physically able to do so, a mother of a hospitalized newborn should begin pumping her milk as soon as possible after the birth and before __ hours after the birth.

    a. 2   c. 12

    b. 6   d. 24

11. Suckling or pumping will cause the greatest rise in blood prolactin concentration

    a. in the daylight morning hours.

    b. in the early afternoon.

    c. in the early evening.

    d. in the hours shortly after midnight.

12. A mother whose baby is unable to feed from the breast should pump about

    a. 8 times in 24 hours around the clock.

    b. 8 times in 24 hours but not necessarily at night.

    c. 5 or 6 times in 24 hours around the clock.

    d. 5 or 6 times in 24 hours but not necessarily at night.

13. The BEST action for a breastfeeding mother who experiences painful engorgement is to

    a. restrict her fluid intake.

    b. use ice packs on her breasts for 20 minutes out of each hour until she is more comfortable.

    c. pump her breasts until milk stops dripping.

    d. work to resolve the engorgement within 48 hours of onset.

14. As compared with large-breasted women, small-breasted women may need to express their breasts

    a. more frequently per 24 hours.

    b. less frequently per 24 hours.

    c. about the same number of times per 24 hours.

    d. by hand rather than with a pump.

15. The highest blood prolactin spikes are produced by

    a. hand expression of one breast at a time.

    b. manual pumping of one breast at a time.

    c. pumping one breast at a time using a hospital-style electric pump.

    d. pumping both breasts at the same time using a hospital-style electric pump.

16. Pumping both breasts at the same time for as long as any milk is extracted usually has what effect on milk fat concentration?

    a. none

    b. slightly increases milk fat concentration

    c. markedly increases milk fat concentration

    d. decreases milk fat concentration somewhat

17. Freshly pumped breastmilk
    a. is sterile.
    b. usually contains only nonpathogenic bacteria.
    c. contains bacteria only if the mother's pumping equipment or technique permits bacterial contamination.
    d. contains bacteria only if the mother herself has a bacterial infection.

18. As compared with healthy full-term infants, compromised preterm infants tolerate
    a. lower concentrations of pathogens in pumped milk, and no nonpathogenic bacteria at all.
    b. lower concentrations of nonpathogenic bacteria in pumped milk, and no pathogens at all.
    c. higher concentrations of pathogens in pumped milk, and no nonpathogenic bacteria at all.
    d. higher concentrations of nonpathogenic bacteria in pumped milk, and no pathogens at all.

19. Pumped breastmilk can be safely stored at ambient temperature (38°C or 100°F) for about
    a. 1 hour.   c. 12 hours.
    b. 4 hours.   d. 24 hours.

20. Pumped breastmilk can be stored in a refrigerator's freezer compartment for a maximum of
    a. 1 week.   c. 2 months.
    b. 2 weeks.   d. 6 months.

21. The nipple soreness that may accompany breast pumping can be reduced by all of the following EXCEPT
    a. using a flange that allows some free space around the nipple.
    b. using a relatively high vacuum setting to shorten the duration of pumping.
    c. eliciting a letdown before applying a vacuum.
    d. switching from one side to the other as milk flow dwindles.

22. A mother with a low milk supply who increases her fluid intake will
    a. usually increase her 24-hour milk yield.
    b. rarely increase her 24-hour milk yield.
    c. usually increase the amount of milk available at any one feeding, but not her 24-hour milk yield.
    d. usually increase the concentration of water-soluble vitamins in her milk.

23. Conditions that may benefit from temporary use of a thin nipple shield include all of the following EXCEPT
    a. flat or inelastic nipples.
    b. baby with a disorganized suck.
    c. small nipple and large infant mouth.
    d. lack of buccal pads in low-birth-weight infant.

24. When a baby is properly positioned over a nipple shield, the baby's lips should be
    a. puckered.
    b. on the flat flange of the shield.
    c. on the firm shaft of the shield.
    d. turned in.

25. The BEST action of a lactation consultant who recommends a nipple shield to a mother is to
    a. document that she recommended a nipple shield.
    b. explain to the mother the risks and benefits of nipple-shield use.
    c. instruct the mother to use the shield at will.
    d. wait at least a week after the mother begins to use a nipple shield to next contact the mother.

26. Milk collected in breast shells between feedings must be discarded because of potential
    a. high concentration of bacteria.
    b. low vitamin concentration.
    c. higher than normal electrolyte concentration.
    d. low concentration of fats.

Discussion Questions

1. In what situations might you consider recommending a nipple shield? In what situations would another alternative be better? What are those alternatives?

2. Should a mother always pump using the maximum negative pressure that a pump will generate? Why or why not? If not, how should she determine the maximum negative pressure to use?

3. What is finger-feeding? When is it appropriate to use? Are there any risks involved in its use?

4. What are the phases of a breast pump cycle? How is each related to the phases of normal infant suckle?

5. Review the instructions accompanying two breast pump kits. Identify information that
    a. is accurate.
    b. is confusing.
    c. improperly describes the lactation process.
    How will your recommendations deal with inaccurate information in these or similar kits?

13

BREASTFEEDING THE PRETERM INFANT

The maternal body is to a degree primed to provide milk for preterm infants, and mother and baby receive physiological and emotional benefits from the act of breastfeeding that far exceed benefits received from the feeding of manufactured milks. Yet mothers of premature infants are among the least likely to breast-feed. Lactation consultants must understand how to help mothers bring in and maintain a milk supply in the absence of a vigorously nursing infant and how to help the infant maximize his breastmilk intake when he does come to the breast. Questions in this chapter will help you to assess your understanding of this body of information and how it applies to professional practice.

Chapter Outline

Maintaining Maternal Milk Volume

    Expressed milk volume guidelines

    Preventing low milk volume

    Skin-to-skin (kangaroo) care

Evidence-Based Guidelines for Milk Collection, Storage, and Feeding

    Guidelines for collection and storage of expressed mothers' milk (EMM)

    Preparing expressed mothers' milk for infant feeding

Special Issues Regarding the Feeding of EMM

    Volume restriction status

    Commercial nutritional additives

    Hindmilk feeding

    Methods of milk delivery

    Maternal medication use

Feeding at Breast in the NICU

    Suckling at the emptied breast

    The science of early breastfeeding

    Progression of in-hospital breastfeeding

    Milk transfer during breastfeeding

Discharge Planning for Postdischarge Breastfeeding

    Getting enough: Determining the need for extra milk feedings

    Methods to deliver extra milk feedings away from the breast

Postdischarge Breastfeeding Management

Summary

Key Concepts

Internet Resources

References

Appendix 13-A: The Preterm Infant Breastfeeding Behavior Scale (PIBBS)

Multiple-Choice Questions

1. Health-care providers should talk about the benefits of breastfeeding preterm infants with
    a. all mothers who deliver preterm infants.
    b. only mothers who deliver preterm infants and who are undecided about breastfeeding.
    c. only mothers who deliver preterm infants and who intend to breastfeed.
    d. only mothers who ask about breastfeeding their preterm infants.

2. In most cases, the mother of a preterm infant will find _____ most effective in obtaining milk.

   a. hand expression

   b. a hand-operated breast pump

   c. an electric breast pump

   d. a battery-operated breast pump

3. Which of the following experiences is NOT considered an inhibitor of prolactin secretion?

   a. prolonged bed rest

   b. delivering a preterm infant

   c. irregular breast emptying

   d. delay in getting the baby to the breast

4. Nonnutritive sucking at the breast usually affects the mother's milk supply by

   a. reducing the amount of milk she is able to pump.

   b. increasing the volume of milk she can pump.

   c. having no particular effect on the volume she can pump.

   d. increasing maternal milk volume only when the baby is about to be released home.

5. As compared with preterm infants fed artificial milks, preterm infants fed human milk experience

   a. decreased intestinal permeability.

   b. delayed motor development during the first year of life.

   c. decreased visual acuity.

   d. decreased rate of gastric emptying.

6. As compared with the milk of a mother of a full-term newborn, the milk of a mother of a 5-day-old premature infant contains higher concentrations of

   a. short-chain fatty acids.

   b. long-chain fatty acids.

   c. iron.

   d. glucose.

7. Preterm mothers' milk typically is not able to sustain optimal

   a. weight gain.

   b. increase in head circumference.

   c. bone mineralization.

   d. metabolic activity.

8. Published studies of mothers' feelings about breastfeeding their preterm infants show that mothers feel that

   a. they have given their infants a good start in life.

   b. the infants preferred being fed breastmilk by bottle to feeding at the breast.

    c. providing breastmilk was inconvenient.

    d. breastfeeding a preterm infant was unpleasant.

9. Around the world, mothers of preterm infants breastfeed at a rate that is

    a. higher than that of the general population.

    b. lower than that of the general population.

    c. higher in industrialized countries but lower in developing countries.

    d. higher in equatorial countries but lower in high-latitude countries.

10. A mother whose preterm baby will not begin enteral feedings for several days should begin expressing fluid from her breasts

    a. as soon after delivery as she is able, to decrease the time until her milk comes in.

    b. a day or so before the baby is expected to begin enteral feeds, so the milk will be fresh.

    c. as soon after delivery as she is able, to obtain colostrum.

    d. when her milk comes in, to avoid breast engorgement.

11. A mother who is able to pump about 800 ml of breastmilk per day for her small, 14-day-old, preterm infant has

    a. fewer alveolar cells in the breast than mothers who pump lesser volumes.

    b. an unnecessarily large milk supply, considering the very small volumes consumed by small preterm infants.

    c. a milk supply large enough to withstand a substantial decline during her infant's hospitalization.

    d. an underlying medical condition causing milk overproduction.

12. When a mother pumps milk from her breasts, she should pump

    a. only until milk stops flowing continuously.

    b. about 15 minutes per breast.

    c. about 15 minutes total on both breasts.

    d. until no more milk droplets appear.

13. The last milk droplets collected contribute most of what component of the milk?

    a. lipids and thus calories

    b. important ions such as Na^+

    c. iron

    d. sugars and thus calories

14. For maximal pumped volumes of breastmilk, a mother should pump

    a. in the relative calm of her own dwelling.

    b. in a "pump room" set aside in the hospital for that purpose.

    c. with a friend at hand for support.

    d. at her infant's bedside.

15. A good rule of thumb for the minimum amount of milk that a mother should be expressing at the time her infant is discharged from the hospital is about

    a. 300 ml/day.   c. 700 ml/day.

    b. 500 ml/day.   d. 1,000 ml/day.

16. Skin-to-skin care ("kangaroo care") can be safely begun with infants

    a. only after they weigh at least 4 pounds, regardless of other medical problems.

    b. only after they weigh at least 4 pounds and have no major medical problems (are "growers").

    c. who are mechanically ventilated, even if they are very small.

    d. once they remain stable in their cribs.

17. Freshly pumped mothers' milk is

    a. sterile.

    b. sterile unless the mother's pumping technique is poor or equipment is contaminated.

    c. usually inoculated only with skin flora.

    d. usually inoculated with large numbers of pathogenic flora and some skin flora.

18. Frozen or refrigerated mothers' milk should be warmed before feeding by

    a. rapid heating (as in a microwave oven) to retain all nutrients.

    b. rapid heating (as in a microwave oven) to retain all immunologic factors.

    c. rapid heating (as in a microwave oven) to retain both nutrients and immunologic factors.

    d. gradual heating to retain both nutrients and immunologic factors.

19. As compared with frozen or chilled breastmilk, fresh breastmilk better helps an infant

    a. grow in length.

    b. resist infection.

    c. resolve nonbreastmilk jaundice.

    d. form blood clots.

20. As compared with premature infants fed manufactured milks, premature infants fed human milk usually

    a. tolerate larger full-volume feedings because the fat content is lower.

    b. tolerate larger full-volume feedings because gastric emptying time is faster.

    c. tolerate smaller full-volume feedings because fat content is higher.

    d. tolerate smaller full-volume feedings because gastric emptying time is slower.

21. Hindmilk and commercial human-milk fortifiers are

    a. interchangeable because both increase the caloric density of human milk.

    b. not interchangeable because hindmilk supplements Ca and P whereas fortifiers add energy.

    c. interchangeable because both promote more rapid growth in the premature infant.

    d. not interchangeable because hindmilk adds energy whereas fortifiers supplement Ca and P.

22. When human milk is fed to a premature infant by gavage, it should be administered by
    a. continuous gavage to avoid straining the capacity of the infant's stomach.
    b. continuous gavage to encourage stable blood concentrations of glucose.
    c. slow intermittent bolus gavage to minimize lipid loss to the gavage tube.
    d. intermittent bolus gavage to help regulate quiet alert states.

23. Lipid-soluble medications used by a breastfeeding mother are composed of molecules that generally
    a. are too large to pass into breastmilk.
    b. are concentrated in foremilk.
    c. are concentrated in hindmilk.
    d. have too short a half-life to be of concern.

24. As compared with premature infants fed by bottle, preterm infants fed at the breast
    a. have a less stable body temperature.
    b. ingest a larger volume of milk.
    c. have less stable oxygenation.
    d. have less interruption in breathing.

25. The optimal frequency of breast pumping in the first week following a premature birth is
    a. 4 to 6 times a day, because that number stimulates the breasts but does not over-tire the mother.
    b. 5 to 7 times in 24 hours, because that number of pumpings means that each pumping session can be shorter.
    c. 6 to 8 times in 24 hours, because that number of pumpings more closely mimics the number of times a healthy term baby would breastfeed.
    d. 8 to 10 times a day, in order to stimulate a large milk supply.

26. The BEST reason for developing a more-than-adequate breastmilk supply at the time an infant is discharged from the hospital is that the extra milk
    a. can be frozen for future use.
    b. will stretch the infant's stomach so he will be able to take larger volumes.
    c. may help to compensate for an infant's weak suck.
    d. ensures good milk ejection when a mother nurses while lying down.

27. As compared with feeding a premature infant directly on the breast, feeding a premature infant through a thin silicone nipple shield
    a. almost always decreases the mother's milk supply.
    b. can allow the infant to ingest larger volumes of milk.
    c. usually causes the infant to bob on and off the breast.
    d. should be pursued no longer than 10 days.

28. During her first few weeks at home, waking a premature infant more than every 3 hours generally is
    a. recommended in order to ensure adequate milk intake to grow.
    b. not recommended in order to avoid hindering the acquisition of state control.

c. recommended in order to ensure adequate hydration.

d. not recommended in order to avoid inhibiting the release of growth hormone.

29. In order to provide her preterm infant with a recognizable benefit, a mother should provide breast fluid for

a. at least one feeding.

b. at least until her milk comes in.

c. at least until her milk fully matures (about 14 days postpartum).

d. at least a month.

30. A mother can attempt to feed a preterm infant at the breast once the infant can

a. reliably maintain her body temperature.

b. consume full bottle-feedings.

c. manage some degree of coordinated sucking and swallowing.

d. stay awake for an entire feeding.

Discussion Questions

1. Why should a milk expression schedule for the mother of a preterm infant parallel the frequency with which a healthy, full-term newborn breastfeeds?

2. How can mothers who pump milk to be fed to their hospitalized infants minimize bacterial contamination of their milk?

3. For optimal breast stimulation, should a mother pump her breasts at the same time or sequentially?

4. Which of the following best indicates that an infant is ready to feed directly from the breast? What is the rationale for your response?

a. The infant can suck rythmically at his mother's soft breast.

b. The infant can take a full bottle of breastmilk.

c. The infant is no longer using supplementary oxygen.

d. The infant has reached 4 pounds in weight.

e. The infant has reached term-corrected age.

5. Are clinical indices of milk intake at the breast adequate for assessing the intake of premature infants? What procedures ensure the validity of test weighing of infants used to determine milk intake?

6. Why are each of the following signs monitored during early breastfeeding sessions for a hospitalized premature infant?

a. heart rate

b. respiratory rate

c. oxygen saturation or transcutaneous oxygen pressure ($TCPO_2$)

d. body temperature

e. test weighing

7. How does the early milk of a mother who delivered a preterm infant differ from the early milk of a mother who delivered a term infant? How long will that difference persist?

8. What is the advantage to the baby of fortifying expressed mother's milk with his own mother's hindmilk? with commercial fortifiers?

9. What is skin-to-skin care (also called kangaroo care)? How does it benefit the infant? How does it benefit the mother?

10. What can be done to make it easier for mothers to pump their milk frequently?

11. How should expressed mother's milk be labeled and stored at home before it is taken to the NICU? in the NICU? How should it be prepared for feeding?

12. What is the relationship between gavage infusion rates and lipid loss? Is lipid loss a problem? What is the rationale for your answer? How can lipid loss be minimized?

13. What pharmaceutical preparations may be recommended to a mother whose milk volumes are faltering? Describe the guidelines for using each.

14

Donor Human Milk Banking

Donor human milk helps to bridge the gap when mother's own milk is not available but an infant does not thrive on manufactured milks. Modern human milk banks balance a humanitarian response to those who require the nutritive or immunological properties of human milk with scrupulous practices to ensure that the donor milk will not cause infection in the recipient. Questions in this chapter will help you to assess your understanding of this body of information and how it applies to professional practice.

Chapter Outline

Multiple-Choice Questions

1. Donor breastmilk obtained directly from another breastfeeding mother is potentially

   a. more healthful than banked milk, because it is fresher (more recently pumped).

   b. less healthful than banked milk, because it cannot be guaranteed to be free of pathogens that cause serious illness.

   c. more healthful than banked milk, because it can be untreated (no heating or freezing), and fresh milk is rarely available from milk banks.

   d. less healthful than banked milk, because the mother may have been in a bad mood when she pumped.

2. In some cultures, banked human milk may be difficult to obtain and dispense because the use of donor milk is generally approved only if

   a. an acquaintance to nurse the baby is not available.

   b. the mother is seriously ill.

   c. a close relative of the recipient infant donates the milk.

   d. the recipient infant will later be wed to a child of the donor.

3. Matching the age of the milk donor's infant with the age of the recipient infant is important because which component changes with time during full lactation in a healthy mother?

   a. sodium content

   b. whey/casein ratio

   c. short-chain/long-chain fatty acid ratio

   d. glucose content

4. Donor milk is most appropriately used in which of the following situations?

   a. Mother has celiac sprue.

   b. Mother is undergoing chemotherapy.

   c. Mother cannot take her baby with her on an extended absence from home.

   d. Mother has a healthy adopted infant.

5. As compared with preterm infants fed manufactured milk, preterm infants fed human milk tend to grow less rapidly, perhaps because
   a. age-appropriate human milk is less calorie dense than manufactured milks.
   b. a greater proportion of human milk is excreted than is metabolized and used for growth.
   c. the volumes of human milk being fed are too small.
   d. human-milk–fed infants are more active and use more calories when they are awake.

6. Pasteurized human milk retains about what proportion IgA, an important immunoglobulin?
   a. about a quarter
   b. about a half
   c. about three-quarters
   d. all of it

7. The incidence of necrotizing entercolitis in premature infants is
   a. increased by early feeds of either artificial milks or human milk.
   b. decreased by early feeds of either artificial milks or human milk.
   c. increased by early feeds of artificial milks but decreased by early feeds of human milk.
   d. decreased by early feeds of artificial milks but increased by early feeds of human milk.

8. The composition of milk of mothers with premature infants differs from the milk of mothers with term infants for about
   a. 1 week.
   b. 2 weeks.
   c. 2 to 4 weeks.
   d. 6 weeks.

9. In most (but not all) countries, mothers who donate their milk are not paid in order to
   a. ensure that donors are highly motivated.
   b. avoid diverting to a bank milk needed to nourish the donor's infant.
   c. avoid the need for bacteriological screening of the milk.
   d. avoid a cost that would be passed along to the recipient's family.

10. Which of the following does NOT disqualify a mother from donating breastmilk?
    a. age below 20
    b. tattoos or body piercings within the previous 12 months
    c. regular use of tobacco
    d. regular use of herbs for medication purposes

11. Which of the following practices is NOT used to guarantee the safety of human milk donors?
    a. heat treatment of all donated milk
    b. screening of potential donors for health history and risk factors
    c. serological screening of potential donors for certain viruses
    d. prevention of donation by mothers whose babies have died

12. Milk banks now rarely use milk obtained by which method?

    a. pumped using a large electric pump

    b. pumped using a manual pump

    c. milk that drips from the breast not being pumped or nursed

    d. expressed by hand

13. The technique known as Holder pasteurization requires that donor milk be held at

    a. 56.5°C for 20 minutes.   c. 56.5°C for 40 minutes.

    b. 62.5°C for 30 minutes   d. 62.5°C for 50 minutes

14. As the temperature of treatment increases, what generally happens to the milk components?

    a. No changes in amounts or proportions of components have been noted.

    b. An increasing proportion of components are inactivated.

    c. A decreasing proportion of components are inactivated.

    d. Immunoglobulins are relatively unaffected, but nutrients progressively are inactivated.

15. Holder pasteurization inactivates

    a. HIV but not cytomegalovirus.

    b. cytomegalovirus but not HIV.

    c. both cytomegalovirus and HIV.

    d. neither cytomegalovirus nor HIV.

16. The World Health Organization and UNICEF jointly propose that, where mother's own milk is not available, the next best choice is

    a. an age-appropriate artificial milk.

    b. donor milk if it is available, or a healthy wet nurse if it is not.

    c. culturally traditional gruels.

    d. diluted whole milk.

17. Small per-bottle fees charged per bottle of donor milk cover the cost of

    a. shipping, screening donors, and the milk itself.

    b. screening donors, the milk itself, and pasteurization.

    c. the milk itself, pasteurization, and shipping.

    d. pasteurization, shipping, and screening donors.

18. Freshly pumped breastmilk can be safely stored at room temperature (about 25°C or 77°F) for no more than

    a. 1 hour.   c. 4 hours.

    b. 2 hours.   d. 6 hours.

19. Thawed frozen breastmilk should be used within

    a. 4 hours.   c. 12 hours.

    b. 8 hours.   d. 24 hours.

20. Frozen human milk is best thawed

    a. in a microwave oven.

    b. in hot water.

    c. in lukewarm water.

    d. on the counter.

21. Unused milk that has been thawed and warmed for a feeding should be

    a. returned to the freezer with a new "freeze date" on the package.

    b. placed in the refrigerator for use within 24 hours.

    c. placed in the refrigerator for use at the next feeding.

    d. discarded as unsuitable for another feeding.

22. The nutrient content of donor milk can be better aligned with the needs of a particular infant by

    a. matching the age of the donor's infant with the age of the recipient infant.

    b. matching the age of the donor with the age of the recipient infant's mother.

    c. pooling analyzed aliquots of milk so that the pooled milk has specified concentrations of protein or fats.

    d. adding infant formula to the milk.

23. In the World Health Organization hierarchy of foods for young infants, the first choice is always

    a. a manufactured milk with denatured proteins.

    b. donor breastmilk.

    c. mother's breastmilk.

    d. gruel or other culturally traditional food.

24. Donor milk is least likely to benefit

    a. premature infants whose own mother's milk supply failed.

    b. toddlers who are highly allergic to table foods.

    c. children who are healing broken bones.

    d. adults preparing to receive a transplanted organ.

Discussion Questions

1. Are recipients of donor breastmilk apt to experience a graft-versus-host reaction? Why or why not?

2. Why do most milk banks process and store donated milk in pooled batches? Provide at least two rationales.

3. How does the Human Milk Banking Association of North America affect the establishment or operation of a milk bank?

4. Are there cultural beliefs that encourage the use of donor breastmilk for an unrelated infant? that discourage the use of donor breastmilk for an unrelated infant? Give specific examples.

5. What is drip milk? Do milk banks currently accept donations of drip milk? Why or why not?

6. For what medical indications might donor milk be prescribed for an infant in a neonatal intensive care unit?

7. Why is the goal to handle donor milk as few times as possible between the donor mother and the recipient infant?

8. What are at least five conditions or practices that will cause a milk bank to decline a person as a donor? Are these conditions or practices temporary or permanent?

9. How has the advent of a widespread incidence of HIV infection affected human milk banking?

BEYOND POSTPARTUM

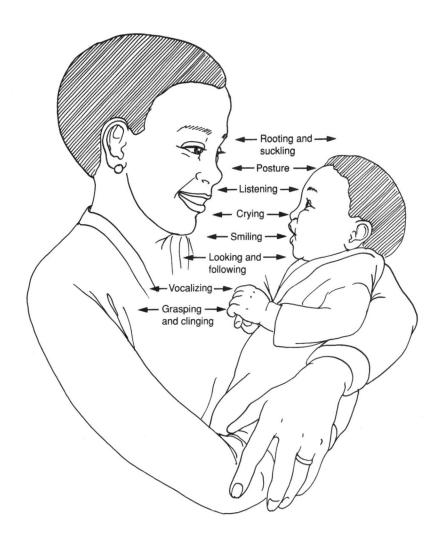

15

Maternal Nutrition During Lactation

Does a mother's diet make a difference to how much breastmilk she produces? Or to her breastmilk's nutritional adequacy? Or to her baby's response to it? The answer is "Probably not–but maybe." Although daily diet usually has little influence on milk composition, some dietary practices–such as strict veganism or rapid weight loss–do. Questions in this chapter will help you to assess your understanding of this body of information and how it applies to professional practice.

Chapter Outline

Maternal Caloric Needs

Maternal Fluid Needs

Weight Loss

Exercise

Calcium Needs and Bone Loss

Vegetarian Diets

Dietary Supplements

Foods that Pass Into Milk

    Caffeine

    Food flavorings

Allergens in Breastmilk

The Goal of the Maternal Diet During Lactation

Nutrition Basics

    Energy

Multiple-Choice Questions

1. What is the effect of a mother's nutritional status on milk volume and composition? Mother's nutritional status has

   a. no effect.

   b. a slight effect.

   c. a moderate to large effect.

   d. a moderate effect before 6 weeks but no effect thereafter.

2. To ensure her own health and maintain adequate milk production, a lactating mother should ingest about how many calories more than her normal prepregnancy intake?

   a. 200   c. 800

   b. 500   d. 1,000

3. About what percentage of food energy is converted to breastmilk?

   a. 40   c. 80

   b. 60   d. 95

4. In order to sustain adequate milk production, a lactating mother should drink

   a. only treated water.

   b. very large quantities of fluid.

   c. to quench her own thirst.

   d. only in between meals.

5. Early signs of dehydration in a lactating mother are

   a. diarrhea and dark yellow urine.

   b. constipation and dark yellow urine.

   c. diarrhea and pale yellow urine.

   d. constipation and pale yellow urine.

6. As compared with mothers who feed artificial milks to their infants, breastfeeding mothers in the first year postpartum tend to

   a. lose more weight.

   b. lose less weight.

   c. lose about the same amount of weight.

   d. lose more weight but only in the first 3 or 4 months.

7. The most rapid rate of weight loss that does not harm milk composition or volume is about 1 kilogram (2.2 pounds)

   a. per month.

   b. per two weeks.

   c. per week.

   d. every other day.

8. Which of the following calorie intakes is the lowest intake that is unlikely to reduce milk volumes in well-nourished women?

   a. 2,600 kcal/day   c. 1,500 kcal/day

   b. 2,200 kcal/day   d. 1,000 kcal/day

9. Extremely rapid maternal weight loss may lead to

   a. a shift of environmental toxins from body fat to breastmilk.

   b. increased rate of infant weight gain as fat shifts into the milk.

   c. stimulation of leaky junctions between lactocytes.

   d. decreased infant weight gain because of decreased protein content of breastmilk.

10. Moderate exercise (but not exercising to exhaustion) by lactating women has been shown to

   a. increase fat content of breastmilk.

   b. decrease milk volume.

   c. decrease lactose content of breastmilk.

   d. increase milk volume.

11. A healthy breastfeeding mother typically experiences a

   a. slight increase of bone density (above prebreastfeeding levels) during the lactational interval.

   b. slight decrease of bone density (below prebreastfeeding levels) following weaning.

   c. greater risk of hip fracture later in life.

   d. lesser risk of hip fracture later in life.

12. How is the calcium intake of a breastfeeding mother related to the calcium content of her milk?

   a. to a moderate degree

   b. to a large degree if she takes calcium supplements

    c. to a large degree if she obtains all calcium from foods

    d. not at all

13. Women who consume a diet devoid of meat, poultry, and dairy products may produce milk that is deficient in

    a. calcium, lactose, and magnesium.

    b. lactose, magnesium, and B_{12}.

    c. magnesium, B_{12}, and calcium.

    d. B_{12}, calcium, and lactose.

14. As of 2004, the Women, Infants, and Children program of the US Department of Health provides food supplements to qualifying low-income lactating mothers for

    a. 3 months.   c. 9 months.

    b. 6 months.   d. 12 months.

15. Mothers of healthy term infants can consume what amount of caffeine without affecting their infants?

    a. none whatsoever

    b. a very small amount

    c. a moderate amount

    d. a large amount

16. Intensely flavored or spicy foods ingested by a lactating woman

    a. rarely impart even a slight flavor to breastmilk.

    b. are the cause of most "nursing strikes."

    c. can expose breastfed infants to pharmacologic concentrations of some compounds.

    d. can prepare an infant to more easily accept table foods.

17. The most common food ingested by lactating women that produces an allergic response in their infants is

    a. citrus fruit.

    b. dairy products.

    c. peanuts.

    d. wheat.

18. The essential amino acids that are required for protein synthesis

    a. are manufactured in the body.

    b. can be obtained only from animal foods.

    c. can be obtained from animal and vegetable sources.

    d. can be obtained only from mixing vegetable sources.

19. Of all the components of breastmilk, the component that most closely reflects the mother's dietary intake is

    a. carbohydrates.

    b. protein.

    c. fats.

    d. vitamins.

20. The main source of energy for all of a lactating woman's body functions is/are

    a. protein.

    b. fats.

    c. carbohydrates.

    d. thyroxine.

21. Vitamins are substances used by the body in very small amounts that

    a. are inorganic.

    b. are heat-generating.

    c. are fat soluble only.

    d. may be stored for long periods or only briefly.

22. Alcohol ingested by a lactating woman

    a. does not enter into breastmilk.

    b. does enter into breastmilk but only in very small amounts.

    c. enters into breastmilk in proportion to the amount consumed.

    d. is rendered inactive in the infant's digestive tract.

23. A lactating woman who intends to consume alcohol should

    a. take no special precautions because alcohol is rendered harmless in the infant's stomach.

    b. take no special precautions because little alcohol crosses into breastmilk.

    c. consume alcohol on an empty stomach so it will metabolize faster.

    d. consume small amounts along with other foods so it will metabolize slowly.

Discussion Questions

1. How is it that a breastfeeding woman needs so few additional calories to support breastmilk production?

2. What would you advise a mother who wishes to begin a weight loss program when her baby is 4 weeks old?

3. Can exercise affect the lactating mother? In what ways? How can such exercise affect the breastfeeding baby?

4. What are three main kinds of vegetarian diets? Do any of them compromise the health of a breastfeeding infant? In what way? How can any deficiency be corrected?

5. What is the effect of a woman drinking several (say, five) cups of coffee a day on her breastfeeding infant? Does the woman need to cut down or cut out her coffee consumption? Does the same hold true if the infant is premature?

6. What are micronutrients? Name three and describe the effect on an infant of a deficiency in each.

7. Does breastfeeding contribute to later osteoporosis in women? What is the rationale for your response?

8. Are multivitamin pills or other vitamin supplements necessary for a breastfeeding mother?

9. Does maternal ingestion of highly flavored foods irritate her breastfeeding infant? Should a lactating woman's own diet be bland? What is the rationale for your response?

10. Do teenage breastfeeding mothers require different nutritional guidelines than do older breastfeeding mothers? What is the rationale for your response?

11. What is the relationship between intensity of exercise and infant refusal to breastfeed? Does this mean lactating women can't exercise at all? What is the rationale for your answer?

16

WOMEN'S HEALTH AND BREASTFEEDING

When a breastfeeding mother is ill–whether the illness is acute or chronic–several questions must be answered: What is the effect of the illness on breastfeeding? What is the effect of breastfeeding on the illness? What will be the physiological and the psychological effects if the baby is weaned in response to his mother's illness? If breastfeeding continues, how can the baby be nourished and protected in the face of his mother's illness? Questions in this chapter will help you to assess your understanding of this body of information and how it applies to professional practice.

Chapter Outline

Alterations in Endocrine and Metabolic Functioning

Diabetes

Thyroid disease

Pituitary dysfunction

Polycystic ovarian syndrome

Theca lutein cysts

Cystic fibrosis

Acute Illness and Infections

Tuberculosis

Group B streptococcus

Dysfunctional uterine bleeding

Maternal Immunizations

Surgery

Donating Blood

Relactation

Induced Lactation

    Domperidone, metoclopramide, and sulpride

Autoimmune Diseases

    Systemic lupus erythematosus

    Multiple sclerosis

    Rheumatoid arthritis

Physically Challenged Mothers

    Seizure disorders

Headaches

Postpartum Depression

    Clinical implications

    Medicines and herbal therapy for depression

    Support for the mother with postpartum depression

Asthma

Smoking

Poison Ivy Dermatitis

Diagnostic Studies Using Radioisotopes

The Impact of Maternal Illness and Hospitalization

Summary

Key Concepts

Internet Resources

References

Multiple-Choice Questions

1. Which of the following maternal conditions is likely to contribute to poor weight gain in the baby?
   a. hypothyroidism
   b. hyperthyroidism
   c. diabetes mellitus
   d. prolactinoma

2. Women in whom gestational diabetes develops during pregnancy should
   a. breastfeed because they will lose weight more rapidly postpartum.
   b. breastfeed because it reduces the risk of type 2 diabetes developing later on.
   c. not breastfeed because lactation impairs maternal glucose metabolism.
   d. not breastfeed because of the risk of mastitis.

3. As compared with healthy, nondiabetic women, women with type 1 diabetes experience lactogenesis II about a day
   a. sooner, because progesterone concentrations are higher.
   b. sooner, because prolactin concentrations are lower.
   c. later, because progesterone concentrations are higher.
   d. later, because prolactin concentrations are lower.

4. After parturition, a diabetic mother excretes in her urine both
   a. lactose and glucose.
   b. lactose and fructose.
   c. glucose and sucrose.
   d. sucrose and fructose.

5. As compared with diabetic mothers who do not breastfeed, diabetic mothers who do breastfeed have average blood glucose concentrations that are
   a. somewhat higher.
   b. about the same.
   c. very slightly lower.
   d. significantly lower.

6. Women with diabetes who breastfeed
   a. may be at greater risk for mastitis than are other breastfeeding women.
   b. may be at less risk for candidiasis than are other breastfeeding women.
   c. will likely need to take more insulin than they did during pregnancy.
   d. should withhold colostrum from their infants until their own blood sugar has stabilized.

7. A diabetic mother who is ready to wean her infant should
   a. wean rapidly, because it's better to deal with the change to her body during only a short interval.
   b. wean rapidly, because then she can enjoy an interval of high calorie intake.
   c. wean slowly, because she can then gradually decrease her own food intake.
   d. wean slowly, because she can then gradually decrease her insulin dosage.

8. A mother who presents with low milk supply, poor infant growth, constantly feeling cold, and thin hair may have
   a. diminished thyroid secretion.
   b. diminished prolactin secretion.
   c. excess thyroid secretion.
   d. excess prolactin secretion.

9. Severe postpartum hemorrhage can result in
   a. increased blood concentration of gonadotropins.
   b. injury to the pituitary that leads to lactation failure.

    c. injury to the hypothalamus, which leads to lactation failure.

    d. injury to the pituitary, which leads to excessive milk production.

10. Breastfeeding can help to reduce postpartum blood loss in the mother because suckling

    a. stimulates the production of clotting factors.

    b. increases the viscosity of the blood.

    c. stimulates release of oxytocin.

    d. decreases the diameter of small blood vessels.

11. When a woman has cystic fibrosis, she

    a. can breastfeed without taking any special measures.

    b. should not breastfeed because she will produce calorie-deficient milk.

    c. should be encouraged to breastfeed despite lipid differences in her milk.

    d. should not breastfeed because of the bacterial pathogens she carries.

12. When a mother has cystic fibrosis, breastfeeding can continue if the mother

    a. loses weight rapidly.

    b. remains in stable health.

    c. increases her vitamin D supplements.

    d. alternates breastmilk feeds with artificial milk feeds.

13. A breastfeeding mother who contracts an acute contagious infection, such as pneumonia, should

    a. temporarily wean to avoid exposing her infant to her illness.

    b. temporarily wean to avoid exposing her infant to the medications used to combat her illness.

    c. continue breastfeeding because the medication that the mother uses will pass to the infant in a therapeutic dosage.

    d. continue breastfeeding in order to pass antibodies to the infant.

14. When a mother has tuberculosis, she

    a. should not breastfeed to avoid contact infection of her infant.

    b. cannot breastfeed her infant because her milk volumes will be small.

    c. may breastfeed her infant after she is treated.

    d. should not breastfeed to avoid infecting her infant through the milk.

15. When a mother must have surgery, she should be encouraged to

    a. breastfeed as late before and as soon after surgery as possible.

    b. begin pumping her breasts 12 hours before surgery and continue for 36 hours afterwards.

    c. breastfeed before the surgery and then pump her breasts for the first week postsurgery.

    d. wean the baby in advance of the surgery to make her life less stressful.

16. A lactating woman may donate blood if the donation takes place at least how many weeks after an uncomplicated birth?

    a. 2   c. 12

    b. 6   d. 20

17. The creation and maintenance of the hormonal milieu required for synthesis of breastmilk requires

    a. functional ovaries.

    b. a preceding pregnancy, even if not full term.

    c. nipple stimulation.

    d. a functional uterus.

18. Domperidone, metoclopramide, and sulpiride are examples of

    a. galactagogues.

    b. analgesics.

    c. milk suppressants.

    d. tranquilizers.

19. The stools of an infant being successfully re-established at the breast after some time being fed manufactured milks will develop

    a. an increasingly unpleasant odor.

    b. a firmer consistency.

    c. a lighter, more yellow color.

    d. a marked increase in volume.

20. The volume of milk synthesized by an adoptive mother without a previous pregnancy depends PRIMARILY on

    a. the vigor with which the infant nurses.

    b. whether the mother has functioning ovaries.

    c. how motivated the mother is.

    d. how long she is able to pump her breasts before the baby arrives.

21. Breastfeeding by a mother with multiple sclerosis (MS), a progressive degenerative neurological disorder, should be

    a. encouraged because something in her milk may protect the infant from later developing MS.

    b. discouraged because of the physical demands it places on her body.

    c. encouraged because it extends the remission of symptoms experienced during pregnancy.

    d. discouraged because the medication commonly prescribed is considered risky for the infant.

22. A mother who experiences postpartum depression is likely to be a

    a. breastfeeding mother who would prefer to bottle-feed.

    b. a bottle-feeding mother who would prefer to breastfeed.

    c. a mother experiencing high levels of stress with few supportive relationships.

    d. a mother who is overly sensitive to hormonal changes after parturition.

23. St. John's wort is an herbal remedy that may be useful in correcting

    a. low milk supply.

    b. overabundant milk supply.

    c. minor depression.

    d. major depression.

24. A mother using medications to control her asthma should be

    a. discouraged from breastfeeding because her medications pose a risk to the infant.

    b. encouraged to breastfeed because it may help protect her infant from asthma.

    c. discouraged from breastfeeding because of the energy drain on her system.

    d. encouraged to breastfeed only if she can discontinue her medications for the duration of breastfeeding.

25. Maternal cigarette smoking during the course of breastfeeding decreases the

    a. risk of respiratory illness in the infant.

    b. carbon monoxide levels in her infant.

    c. fat content of breastmilk.

    d. risk of maternal breast abscess.

26. Diabetes mellitus is

    a. an acute illness in the breastfeeding baby of the mother with diabetes.

    b. a chronic illness in the mother; she should not be encouraged to breastfeed.

    c. a chronic illness in the mother; she should be encouraged to breastfeed.

    d. a chronic illness in the breastfeeding baby of the mother with diabetes.

27. Postpartum changes in a diabetic woman's blood glucose concentrations

    a. are of no particular concern with respect to breastfeeding.

    b. produce maternal hypoglycemia in the first few hours after birth.

    c. produce maternal hyperglycemia in the first few hours after birth.

    d. cause urine to excrete more lactose than usual around day three postpartum.

28. Replacement insulin taken by a diabetic mother does not affect her breastfeeding infant because the insulin molecule is

    a. inactived by acid in the infant's stomach.

    b. transferred to the infant in dosages that are only a small proportion of his own insulin production.

    c. too alkaline to pass into breastmilk.

    d. too large to pass into breastmilk.

29. If her mother smokes cigarettes daily, the infant is better off being fed
    a. manufactured milk, to avoid ingesting nicotine-containing breastmilk.
    b. at the breast, to obtain the immunological protection of human milk.
    c. manufactured milk, to avoid being handled by a mother whose hands are frequently at her mouth.
    d. at the breast, because nicotine is inert in the infant's system.

30. A nursing mother who develops a contact dermatitis from poison ivy should
    a. discontinue breastfeeding until her skin heals.
    b. discontinue breastfeeding because breastfeeding will exacerbate her discomfort.
    c. continue breastfeeding but prevent the baby's mouth from touching the lesions.
    d. continue breastfeeding without restrictions.

31. The length of time that a mother treated with radioactive isotopes must avoid breastfeeding her infant is shortened by
    a. using an isotope more soluble in breastmilk.
    b. using an isotope with a shorter half-life.
    c. being treated with many smaller dosages rather than one larger one.
    d. pumping the breasts to remove radioactive milk.

32. A breastfeeding mother with epilepsy
    a. is more likely to drop her infant than is a mother with epilepsy who bottle-feeds.
    b. must forgo her treatment regimen during the course of breastfeeding.
    c. can breastfeed if her infant is monitored for drug reactions.
    d. should not consider breastfeeding.

Discussion Questions

1. What is the difference between an acute and a chronic illness? Describe an example of each.

2. What are at least four ways in which a lactating woman can prepare to minimize separation or interruption of breastfeeding caused by her own surgery? by her infant's surgery?

3. How does cigarette smoking affect women, as a group, in their breastfeeding course?

4. What is a prolactinoma? What restrictions does it place on breastfeeding?

5. During a lactating woman's self-limiting acute illness, should she as a general rule interrupt breastfeeding? By continuing to breastfeed, does the infant obtain any benefits? Does the infant incur any risk?

6. Severe postpartum hemorrhage may be associated with what breastfeeding outcome? Describe the physiology causing this outcome.

7. What physiological pathways allow induced lactation (as in the case of an adopted infant) to succeed to some degree? Why then do most adoptive mothers who induce lactation also offer supplements to their infants? What are at least two factors in the mother and two in the infant that may make it difficult for the mother to bring in a full milk supply?

8. How can a physically impaired mother, a mother with a seizure disorder, or a mother with rheumatoid arthritis manage breastfeeding? Is breastfeeding inherently riskier to the baby's safety than bottle-feeding? How do you justify your answer?

9. What is the difference between relactation and induced lactation? What are the potential benefits of each? Are their any potential risks or other downsides?

10. What are three degrees of postpartum depression? Are they affected by the normal postpartum shifts in hormones? Does breastfeeding influence the course of postpartum depression?

11. Does a woman who smokes face any increased health risks related to breastfeeding? Does her infant face any health risks related to her mother's smoking?

12. Can breastfeeding and headache be related? What physiology underlies the connection? What are some suggestions to help the mother cope?

Maternal Employment and Breastfeeding

Maintaining breastfeeding while being employed outside the home isn't particularly easy—but in many circumstances it is possible. A lactation consultant can advise on arrangements concerning the workplace, family (especially sleeping), day care, and pumping that facilitate continued breastfeeding. Questions in this chapter will help you to assess your understanding of this body of information and how it applies to professional practice.

Chapter Outline

Multiple-Choice Questions

1. Mothers who express breastmilk at their place of employment
   a. are more likely to miss work because of breast infections.
   b. are more likely to leak milk.
   c. are less likely to miss work because of illness in their infants.
   d. are more susceptible to milk stasis.

2. "Reverse cycle nursing" refers to
   a. a breast pump's cycling pattern that reverses the pressure exerted on the breast.
   b. an infant's pattern of breastfeeding more at night and sleeping more during the day.
   c. breastfeeding on the weekend on the same schedule a mother uses when she is at work.
   d. breastfeeding just to the point of breast comfort to reduce a milk supply so that a mother need not express milk on the job.

3. Job-sharing refers to
   a. one partner employed full time at home and the other employed full time outside the home.
   b. two individuals working part time in the same job.
   c. completing part of one's employment duties at home and part of them in the workplace.
   d. dividing home responsibilities between partners.

4. Research on the effect of maternal paid employment on breastfeeding indicates that
   a. planned return to work does not change the rate of breastfeeding initiation, but it does shorten the overall duration of breastfeeding.
   b. planned return to work lowers both the rate of breastfeeding initiation and overall duration of breastfeeding.
   c. working full time rather than part time lengthens overall breastfeeding duration.
   d. the younger an infant when the mother returns to work, the longer the overall duration of breastfeeding.

5. After it is pumped, the ability of fresh, room-temperature breastmilk to kill bacteria is highest
   a. for about 45 minutes.
   b. for about 2 hours.
   c. for about 6 hours.
   d. for about 12 hours.

6. A portion of thawed breastmilk that remains after a bottle-feeding
   a. should be promptly refrigerated and used at the next feeding.
   b. may be layered on top of still-frozen milk and used as is convenient.
   c. should be discarded.
   d. may be left at room temperature if the next feeding will be within 3 hours.

7. Infants and young children cared for outside their own homes have higher rates of
   a. lower respiratory infections.
   b. gastroesophageal reflux.
   c. infections related to teething.
   d. diarrhea.

8. The percentage of women who combine working and breastfeeding is
   a. higher in less-skilled occupations.
   b. higher in more-skilled occupations.
   c. about the same, regardless of skill level of the occupation.
   d. lowest in mothers who work at home.

9. The International Labour Organization promotes the right of women to
   a. breastfeed in the workplace.
   b. have access to all professions.
   c. be paid wages comparable to those paid men in comparable jobs.
   d. qualify for child subsidies so they may leave the paid workforce during their child-bearing years.

10. Pumped milk that is "layered"–freshly pumped milk added to already frozen milk–should be labeled with
    a. the week in which the milk was pumped.
    b. the date that the first (lowest) portion of milk was pumped.
    c. the date that the last (highest) portion of milk was pumped.
    d. the date on which it is estimated that the milk will be used.

11. Mothers who view breastfeeding positively are inclined to
    a. breastfeed longer, even if they are employed.
    b. select home care settings rather than group day care for their babies.
    c. delay until 6 months their return to work, in order to stay with their babies.
    d. decide not to return to work following their babies' birth.

Discussion Questions

1. Considering the time and effort required to pump breastmilk for their infant, why do mothers continue to do so? What are the advantages to the infant? to the employed mother? to her employer? What are possible disadvantages to the employer?

2. What conditions promote allowing a mother to comfortably breastfeed or pump at her work site?

3. What factors should a mother consider as she arranges day care for her infant? What should the day care provider know about breastfeeding infants? How will milk be offered to the infant? How can the mother tell if the baby has been given manufactured milk feedings without the mother's approval?

4. What illnesses are common in infants placed in day care? What effect does breastfeeding have on the likelihood that the breastfed infant will fall ill?

5. Who are at least three persons whose support may permit a working and breastfeeding mother to continue breastfeeding longer? What do these people do to support continued breastfeeding?

6. Is a longer pumping session necessarily a "better" pumping session, if volume of milk obtained is the criterion? What combination of pumping frequency and duration maximizes the amount of milk that can be pumped in a day?

7. When is an employed mother likely to experience each of the following? How can she minimize each?

   a. engorgement or leaking

   b. the baby's frequent changes of feeding patterns

   c. concern about an inadequate or fluctuating milk supply

   d. the need to express or pump milk

8. What considerations control when a breastfeeding mother returns to paid employment? If the mother has some flexibility, how might she phase back in to her employment?

18

Child Health

How does breastfeeding affect the normal development and health of young children? How do feeding routines change as an infant grows? Questions in this chapter will help you to assess your understanding of this body of information and how it applies to professional practice.

Chapter Outline

Solid Foods
    Introducing solid foods
    Choosing the diet
    Choosing feeding location
    Delaying solid foods
Obesity
Co-Sleeping
Long-Term Breastfeeding
Weaning
Implications for Practice
Summary
Key Concepts
Internet Resources
References

Multiple-Choice Questions

1. Studies of cognitive ability tend to show that, as compared with infants fed manufactured milks, breast-fed infants

    a. score higher around the world.

    b. score lower around the world.

    c. score about the same around the world.

    d. score higher in developing regions of the world but about the same in industrialized nations.

2. Motor development in a child progresses from

    a. small muscle control to large muscle control.

    b. feet and legs to arms and head.

    c. large muscle control to small muscle control.

    d. trunk first, then legs, then arms.

3. As compared with his birth weight and length, a year-old baby has on average

    a. doubled both weight and length.

    b. doubled weight and increased length by half.

    c. tripled weight and doubled length.

    d. tripled weight and increased length by half.

4. As compared with infants fed manufactured milks, the growth in head circumference of breastfed infants is

    a. faster.

    b. about the same.

    c. slower.

    d. faster during the first 4 to 6 months but about the same thereafter.

5. As compared with never-breastfed infants, during their first 8 months breastfed infants usually weigh

    a. slightly more during the entire interval.

    b. somewhat less during the entire interval.

    c. about the same for the first 4 months, but weigh less later.

    d. about the same for about 4 months, but weigh more later.

6. An infant suffering malnutrition first experiences

    a. loss of visual acuity.

    b. decrease in rate of weight gain.

    c. decrease in rate of linear growth.

    d. decrease in rate of growth in head circumference.

7. Which of the following senses are well developed in term neonates?

    a. hearing, smell, and taste

    b. smell, taste, and vision

    c. taste, vision, and hearing

    d. vision, hearing, and smell

8. _____ infants recognize axillary odors of their mothers.

    a. Both breastfed and artificially fed

    b. Neither breastfed nor artificially fed

    c. Only breastfed

    d. Only artificially fed

9. Neonates generally prefer to look at

    a. objects about 10 inches from their face.

    b. objects that display a single solid color.

    c. red objects.

    d. stationary objects on which they can focus.

10. A fully developed, functional central nervous system is indicated in a neonate who

    a. blinks her eyes.

    b. moves rapidly between alert, fussy, and sleep states.

    c. coordinates suck and swallow.

    d. has a strong startle reflex.

11. The infant can best maintain complex interactions with his environment in the

    a. drowsy state.

    b. quiet awake state.

   c. alert, inactive state.

   d. fussing state.

12. As compared with infants fed manufactured milks, breastfed infants usually sleep

   a. more in the late afternoon and early evening.

   b. later in the morning.

   c. shorter intervals at night.

   d. longer intervals at night.

13. With respect to social interactions, neonates are

   a. passive, responding only to caregiver cues.

   b. passive, responding only to their own internal needs.

   c. active, but unfocused in interactions with caregivers.

   d. active, initiating desired responses by the caregiver.

14. The end of a particular feeding bout is more apt to be decided by

   a. the infant, if the baby is breastfed.

   b. the mother, if the baby is breastfed.

   c. the mother and baby jointly, if the infant is breastfed.

   d. the baby, if the baby is bottle-fed.

15. Early neonatal exposure to rubella virus in breastmilk

   a. is likely to be harmful to the infant.

   b. strengthens the response to later rubella vaccination in the infant.

   c. does not alter the response to later rubella vaccination in the infant.

   d. diminishes the response to later rubella vaccination in the infant.

16. As compared with infants fed manufactured milks, immunization of breastfed children

   a. should be delayed until after weaning to assure that the immunization "takes."

   b. usually results in a higher antibody concentration.

   c. should be on a different schedule.

   d. should be avoided in order to avoid a possible adverse reaction to the immunization medium.

17. The American Academy of Pediatrics does not routinely recommend vitamin supplements for breast-fed infants with the exception of

   a. vitamin A.   c. vitamin D.

   b. vitamin C.   d. vitamin E.

18. The likelihood of rickets developing in an infant increases with

   a. darker skin color.

   b. residence closer to the equator.

   c. decreased area of skin covered by clothing.

   d. increased opportunities to be outside.

19. Dental caries in young breastfeeding children are usually associated with
    a. nutritional deficiencies in the mother while she was pregnant.
    b. night-time breastfeedings.
    c. ear infections.
    d. refined sugars in juices or sodas offered to the child.

20. It is difficult for an infant to ingest soft foods until her tongue-extrusion reflex diminishes, which occurs around age
    a. 6 weeks.   c. 6 months.
    b. 3 months.   d. 9 months.

21. The risk of allergies developing in an infant born into an allergic family can be most greatly reduced by
    a. offering no milk other than breastmilk, and waiting 4 months to begin soft table foods.
    b. offering no milk other than breastmilk, and waiting 6 months to begin soft table foods.
    c. offering no milk other than breastmilk for 4 months, and then offering manufactured milk when soft table foods are introduced.
    d. offering only manufactured milk and introducing soft table foods by 2 months.

22. Offering soft solids, such as cereals, to infants at bedtime generally will
    a. not change the infant's sleep pattern.
    b. increase the time it takes the baby to fall asleep.
    c. markedly reduce night waking.
    d. increase night waking.

23. Babies being introduced to soft table foods accept them more easily if the foods are
    a. mixed with breastmilk.
    b. mixed with water.
    c. highly salted.
    d. cold.

24. Infants of mothers who consume a vegan diet lacking meat, dairy products, and eggs may need to be supplemented with which vitamin?
    a. A   c. B_6
    b. B_1 d. B_{12}

25. The safety of an infant sleeping with his mother is increased if
    a. the baby is placed on his back.
    b. a heated waterbed is shared.
    c. the baby is propped in position with soft blankets or pillows.
    d. the baby is placed on his stomach.

26. A mother who weans rapidly may be more comfortable if she
    a. expresses or pumps her breasts to relieve overfullness.
    b. goes without a brassiere to avoid pressure on the breasts.

   c. takes cold showers to reduce circulation in the breast.

   d. firmly kneads her breasts to break up incipient plugged ducts.

27. As compared with infants fed manufactured milks, breastfed infants

   a. are less wakeful at night.

   b. are more wakeful in the early evening.

   c. are less wakeful in the early evening.

   d. sleep more hours per 24-hour day.

28. As compared with infants fed manufactured milks, breastfed infants are

   a. less likely to have misaligned teeth, but the likelihood of misalignment increases as the duration of breastfeeding increases.

   b. less likely to have misaligned teeth, and the likelihood of misalignment decreases as the duration of breastfeeding increases.

   c. more likely to have misaligned teeth.

   d. about as likely to have misaligned teeth.

29. Children of obese parents are less likely themselves to be obese if they are breastfed because

   a. a factor in breastmilk alters the genes responsible for the tendency to obesity.

   b. breastfed infants regulate their own intake.

   c. breastmilk has a lower caloric density than manufactured milks.

   d. breastfeeding itself uses considerably more calories than does bottle-feeding.

Discussion Questions

1. What are the various states of arousal in an infant? Which state is optimal for breastfeeding? Why is this so?

2. What is the relationship between sleeping with an infant and infant night waking? prolonged breast-feeding? What physiology underlies any advantage to night breastfeeds?

3. What reflexes are present during a healthy infant's first few months? What effect, if any, do they have on breastfeeding?

4. Does the addition of solid foods make a young infant (less than 4 months old) more likely to gain weight more quickly? sleep through the night? Explain the physiology underlying your response.

5. What does the addition of table foods to a 4-month-old infant's diet do to maternal milk volumes? What will happen to milk volumes if solids are delayed until 6 or 7 months?

6. Can breastfeeding toddlers develop tooth decay? Why or why not? What mechanisms are in operation?

The Ill Child: Breastfeeding Implications

Can children breastfeed if they are born with health problems or become ill? Can they be fed breastmilk? Lactation consultants are expected to provide strategies that optimize breastfeeding by the compromised infant and to support the families who must cope with emotionally draining situations. Questions in this chapter will help you to assess your understanding of this body of information and how it applies to professional practice.

Chapter Outline

Multiple-Choice Questions

1. A 3-month-old breastfeeding infant should normally produce how many wet cloth diapers in 24 hours?
   a. two to four.
   b. three to six.
   c. four to seven.
   d. six to eight.

2. Which of the following is one indicator of dehydration?
   a. depressed posterior fontanel
   b. dry mucous membranes
   c. very warm extremities
   d. slower-than-usual pulse

3. A breastfeeding infant who presents with pronounced dehydration resulting from an acute gastrointestinal illness should be fed
   a. only breastmilk.
   b. only oral rehydration solution.
   c. only a soy-based manufactured baby milk.
   d. breastmilk and oral rehydration solution.

4. A good time to try to feed a slow-gaining breastfed infant is when the infant is
   a. sleeping soundly, because she will not then resist.
   b. awake but quiet, because she is most receptive.
   c. is fussing, because she is probably hungry.
   d. is crying, because crying produces a wide gape.

5. Families of infants born with chronic health problems MOST appreciate advice that
   a. is accurate.
   b. is given tactfully out of consideration for the parents' stressful situation.
   c. doesn't focus on possible problems.
   d. is presented abruptly, to get all information on the table.

6. When breastmilk must be fed by hand to a young infant for many weeks, the method that puts the most volume into the infant is
   a. cup-feeding.
   b. finger-feeding.
   c. syringe-feeding.
   d. bottle-feeding.

7. A mother who bottle-feeds her infant can mimic the experience of breastfeeding by
    a. feeding the baby next to her bare breast.
    b. positioning the baby so that the baby faces away from her.
    c. ending the feeding after 10 minutes.
    d. gently introducing the bottle nipple into the infant's mouth.

8. A breastfeeding infant who is a surgical patient should
    a. abstain from breastfeeds for at least 4 hours prior to surgery.
    b. nurse within 3 hours before surgery.
    c. be given a first feeding of glucose water after surgery.
    d. begin breastfeeding as soon as any oral feedings can resume.

9. As compared with an infant fed manufactured milk, a breastfed infant experiences greater
    a. risk of infection, because he is relying on maternal antibodies.
    b. weight loss during an infection-caused illness.
    c. risk of hospitalization.
    d. protection from infection in a dose-dependant manner.

10. Treatment for mild dehydration during gastroenteritis in breastfeeding infants includes
    a. continued breastfeeding and rehydration fluids if needed.
    b. interrupted breastfeeding and breast pumping during the acute phase of the illness while the child receives oral rehydration solutions.
    c. continued breastfeeding and formula supplementation.
    d. hospitalization with intravenous fluids and electrolytes.

11. Excessive fluid loss in an infant with gastroenteritis is most likely due to
    a. vomiting and diarrhea.
    b. increased urination.
    c. increased insensible water loss.
    d. increased perspiration.

12. During gastroenteritis in a breastfed infant, breastfeeding should be interrupted during
    a. the rehydration phase of an illness, but not the recovery phase.
    b. the recovery phase of an illness, but not the rehydration phase.
    c. both the rehydration and the recovery phase.
    d. neither the rehydration nor the recovery phase.

13. An infant with an ear infection or respiratory infection may breastfeed better in which position?
    a. upright
    b. side-lying
    c. football (clutch)
    d. cross-cradle

14. The likelihood of otitis media developing in a breastfed infant can BEST be reduced by
    a. placing her in day care, to help her immune system mature more rapidly.
    b. avoiding tobacco smoke in the home.
    c. limiting night-time feedings.
    d. free use of pacifiers.

15. Excessively low muscle tone can express itself in a young breastfeeding infant by
    a. a complete seal of lips on the breast.
    b. an easily stimulated gag reflex.
    c. generation of little negative pressure during suck.
    d. a breast drawn deeply into the oral space.

16. Excessively high muscle tone can express itself in a young breastfeeding infant as
    a. arching of the back.
    b. a wide gape before latching onto the breast.
    c. breast falling to the back of the infant's mouth.
    d. a cupped tongue.

17. Both hypotonic infants and hypertonic infants are more likely to obtain more milk from the breast if the mother uses
    a. breast shells.
    b. a feeding-tube device at the breast.
    c. timed feedings.
    d. a thin silicone nipple shield.

18. A breastfeeding neonate who has congenital heart disease may
    a. maintain a good pink color.
    b. begin a feeding by suckling vigorously.
    c. nurse at a consistent pace for the entire feeding.
    d. breathe slowly during feedings.

19. The best predictor of duration of any breastfeeding by an infant born with heart defects has been shown to be
    a. the severity of the defect.
    b. the innate breastfeeding ability of the infant.
    c. the birth weight of the infant.
    d. the degree of the mother's determination to continue breastfeeding.

20. A breastfed infant with congenital heart disease is likely to be more comfortable in a feeding position that
    a. hyperextends his neck.
    b. flexes his knees.

    c. extends his hips.

    d. tips his chin down.

21. Breastmilk feedings reduce the risk of otitis media in infants with cleft lip or palate during

    a. the interval of any breastfeeding.

    b. any breastfeeding and beyond weaning.

    c. the interval of exclusive breastfeeding.

    d. about the first 3 months of life.

22. An infant with an unrepaired cleft lip (but no palatal clefts)

    a. is usually uninterested in breastfeeding.

    b. will feed better if swaddled.

    c. develops better suction if placed at breast so that the cleft is always "up."

    d. has ineffective jaw excursions.

23. A child born with a cleft palate when put to the breast commonly will

    a. try to fill the cleft with his tongue.

    b. regurgitate milk into the nostrils.

    c. firmly grasp the breast.

    d. prefer to nurse in a side-lying position.

24. An infant with an unrepaired cleft palate will find breastfeeding easiest in which position?

    a. prone on mother's chest

    b. side-lying

    c. football (clutch)

    d. upright

25. An infant born with a cleft palate can be expected to

    a. gain normally with exclusive breastfeeding, once a good feeding position is determined.

    b. require smaller volumes of breastmilk to meet his metabolic needs.

    c. be at high risk for failure to thrive with exclusive breastfeeding.

    d. obtain little benefit from breastfeeding because milk strays from the oral cavity during nursing.

26. Infants with Pierre Robin sequence feed poorly in the early weeks because

    a. they have a tonic bite.

    b. they cannot take enough breast tissue into the mouth.

    c. they have overly long jaw excursions.

    d. they cannot rhythmically swallow the milk drawn from the breast.

27. Breastfed infants who experience continual gastroesophageal reflux (constantly spit up large quantities)

    a. should be monitored for adequate growth.

    b. may be signaling readiness for solid foods.

    c. will cough less if breastmilk is thickened with cereal.

    d. usually have the same problem as older children.

28. To maximally reduce the phenylalanine load in infants born with phenylketonuria, such infants should

    a. breastfeed exclusively.

    b. be fed solely a low-phenylalanine manufactured baby milk.

    c. combine breastmilk with phenylalanine-free manufactured baby milk.

    d. combine standard formula and phenylalanine-free manufactured baby milk feedings.

29. Which of the following conditions in an infant contraindicates all breastfeeding?

    a. galactosemia

    b. cystic fibrosis

    c. phenylketonuria

    d. celiac disease

30. Jaundice in newborns may result from all of the following EXCEPT

    a. rapid hemolysis.

    b. type 1 diabetes.

    c. galactosemia.

    d. hypothyroidism.

31. Celiac disease in an infant is best managed by

    a. breastfeeding exclusively only briefly and early introduction of milk supplements and solids.

    b. breastfeeding exclusively only briefly, early introduction of milk supplements, and late introduction of solids.

    c. breastfeeding as long as possible combined with early introduction of solids.

    d. breastfeeding as long as possible and late introduction of solids.

32. As compared with manufactured milks, breastmilk promotes growth of infants born with cystic fibrosis because

    a. it spends a longer time in the infant's stomach, thus more nutrients can be absorbed.

    b. it contains larger amounts of milk lipase, which aids the absorption of fats.

    c. it increases the infant's appetite, so a greater volume of milk is consumed.

    d. it promotes absorption of vitamins B and C, which increase growth rate.

33. Neonates who show no adverse reaction to a feeding of bovine-based milk in the nursery in the first 3 days of life

    a. will never be allergic to bovine milk.

    b. are too young to develop allergic reactions.

    c. may express allergic symptoms if they ingest bovine-based milk later.

    d. will not develop any allergic reaction now or later if all subsequent feeds are bovine-based milk.

34. Allergic reactions in an exclusively breastfed baby are most likely
    a. to the breastmilk itself.
    b. caused by foreign proteins in the breastmilk.
    c. caused by fats in the breastmilk.
    d. caused by inhalants or topical substances.

35. Transient lactase deficiency in an infant's intestinal brush border may lead to diarrhea after the infant has
    a. experienced upper respiratory illness.
    b. experienced lower respiratory illness.
    c. been prescribed analgesics.
    d. fed on both breasts of a mother with an abundant milk supply.

36. Feeding an infant with Down syndrome may be complicated by
    a. strong peristalsis of the tongue.
    b. hypotonicity of the oral muscles.
    c. associated problems of glucose transport.
    d. tongue fixed to the roof of the mouth.

Discussion Questions

1. How might a mother who suspects family allergies to certain foods or groups of foods reduce the risk of atopic illness in a subsequent child? What can she do before the new baby is born? after the baby is born?

2. What is the difference between food allergy, food sensitivity, and food intolerance? How does breast-feeding affect each?

3. What are five foods that are associated with allergic reactions in infants and young children? What is the offending molecule in the food?

4. What are advantages—to the infant, family, and health-care system—of early repair of cleft lip?

5. What is the relationship between breastfeeding and upper respiratory infection in infants? breastfeeding and lower respiratory infection? What accounts for any difference?

6. What illnesses are contraindications to exclusive breastfeeding or to even partial breastfeeding? What physiology underlies these illnesses?

7. As compared with the presurgery fasting period for infants fed manufactured milks, how long is the fasting period—both before and after surgery—for a breastfed infant? How can a mother comfort her infant during this fasting interval?

8. How do each of the following conditions affect oral feedings in general and breastfeeding in particular?

    a. choanal atresia

    b. cleft palate

    c. tracheoesophageal fistula

    d. pyloric stenosis

    e. imperforate anus

    f. esophageal reflux

9. What main points would you make to emergency-room staff who must care for a breastfeeding mother or a breastfeeding infant admitted for care?

10. How would you help a breastfeeding mother, physically and emotionally, whose young infant has died?

20

Infant Assessment

The new baby's contribution to bringing in his mother's milk supply cannot be overemphasized. An evaluation of the infant's motor abilities, reflexes, and neurobehavioral states will suggest specific strategies for the lactation consultant to use as she helps the mother initiate breastfeeding. Questions in this chapter will help you to assess your understanding of this body of information and how it applies to professional practice.

Chapter Outline

Multiple-Choice Questions

1. A term infant is one born during
   a. 36 through 40 weeks gestation.
   b. 37 through 40 weeks gestation.
   c. 37 through 41 weeks gestation.
   d. 38 through 42 weeks gestation.

2. A tool commonly used to assess gestational age (New Ballard Score) relies on
   a. neither physical nor neurological characteristics.
   b. physical characteristics alone.
   c. neurological characteristics alone.
   d. both physical and neurological characteristics.

3. Audible swallowing by a neonate who is at the breast indicates that
   a. the baby is less than about 3 days old.
   b. lactogenesis I has occurred.
   c. milk likely is being transferred.
   d. the baby has an aberrant tongue position.

4. An infant who is rooting typically
   a. turns her head toward a stimulus.
   b. lifts her tongue to the roof of her mouth.

    c. purses her lips.

    d. makes licking movements.

5. An infant who is latched on firmly to the breast

    a. is probably creasing his mother's nipple.

    b. has his lower lip turned in.

    c. retains the breast during pauses in nursing.

    d. has a tonic bite.

6. During swallowing, an infant at the breast also

    a. retracts her cheeks.

    b. depresses the back of the tongue.

    c. flares her nares.

    d. drops and then raises her lower jaw.

7. Putting a baby to breast during the first hour postpartum usually is

    a. a good move, because the baby (if unmedicated) is alert and responsive.

    b. a poor move, because the baby needs to recover from the delivery and shouldn't be expending more energy.

    c. not necessary, because the baby will shortly fall into a deep sleep and doesn't need the calories.

    d. a good move, because it will speed up the time at which lactogenesis II occurs.

8. Most newborns have passed the first meconium stool within the first _____ hours after birth.

    a. 4   c. 16

    b. 8   d. 24

9. Vernix caseosa, a secretion on the skin surface, is usually

    a. visible on term infants.

    b. not visible on term infants.

    c. a sign of a stressful labor and delivery.

    d. more pronounced on postterm infants.

10. Neonatal skin that quickly returns to its original shape after being gently pinched may indicate

    a. excessive fetal weight gain in the third trimester.

    b. adequate interstitial fluid in the skin.

    c. that the infant requires more fluids.

    d. inadequate fetal weight gain in the third trimester.

11. A young infant's anterior fontanel

    a. depresses when the infant coughs.

    b. is sunken when the infant is dehydrated.

    c. closes between 2 and 3 months of age.

    d. has a triangular shape.

12. A neonate's visual abilities enable him to
    a. focus on objects around 24 inches (60 cm) from his eyes.
    b. follow to the midline objects that move.
    c. converge his eyes.
    d. respond to stationary more than to moving objects.

13. In a healthy term neonate, a familiar voice will elicit
    a. an eyeblink.
    b. immediate initiation or increase in body movement.
    c. a gaze that remains fixed in the direction it held before the voice was heard.
    d. wrinkling of the brow.

14. The nose of a term newborn
    a. cannot be compressed on either side (on one naris) without compromising the infant's airway.
    b. drains mucus for the first few days after birth.
    c. contains enough cartilage that it rarely displays asymmetry from intrauterine compression.
    d. may be the terminus of a cleft lip or palate.

15. The mouth of a healthy term neonate contains
    a. thin buccal pads that are ready to grow as breastfeeding progresses.
    b. relatively dry mucous membranes that give more traction to hold the breast in the mouth.
    c. a tongue that fits easily behind the gumline when the mouth is closed.
    d. a gum ridge that contains the tongue when the mouth is open.

16. A tight lingual frenulum may be associated with
    a. a heart-shaped indentation in the tip of the tongue.
    b. inability of the infant to gape widely.
    c. a short upper lip.
    d. extremely short jaw excursions during breastfeeding.

17. A healthy term neonate's palate should
    a. be smooth and contain a high central "bubble."
    b. be gently arched with a small cleft in the soft palate.
    c. be smooth, gently arched, and intact.
    d. contain pronounced rugae to help hold the breast in place.

18. An infant whose chest retracts during breathing
    a. is overly hungry and needs to be put to the breast.
    b. is working to breathe and is unlikely to breastfeed well.
    c. is overly excited and is better fed by bottle.
    d. is working to breathe and likely will settle down once at the breast.

19. In the first week postpartum, pink or red stains in the diaper owing to uric acid crystals are a consequence of

    a. excessive breastmilk.

    b. bovine milk.

    c. soy milk.

    d. poor hydration.

20. During the first week, a breastfed newborn's stools progress in color as follows:

    a. black, greenish brown, green.

    b. greenish black, tan, brown.

    c. black, greenish brown, mustard.

    d. brownish black, yellow, green.

21. The sleep wake states in which a newborn breastfeeds most effectively are

    a. quiet sleep, drowsy.

    b. deep sleep, quiet alert.

    c. quiet alert, active alert.

    d. drowsy, quiet alert.

22. A newborn who grimaces and arches is

    a. hungry and ready to feed.

    b. overstimulated and needs rest.

    c. energetic and ready to interact with others.

    d. sleepy and ready for the crib.

23. On day one or two of life, a newborn who refuses to nurse on a particular breast is likely to be

    a. guarding against pain exacerbated when positioned at the refused breast.

    b. conserving her energy until her mother's milk comes in.

    c. aware that the refused breast is infected.

    d. displaying a random notion that will disappear shortly.

Discussion Questions

1. Describe the normal range of vital signs (temperature, pulse, respirations) in a newborn.

2. Describe three features of infant anatomy that are directly related to the neonate's ability to suckle. How could early assessment of these features help prevent breastfeeding failure?

3. Name three breastfeeding assessment tools. Which tool do you think is best to use in clinical practice? Why?

4. Make a physical assessment of a breastfeeding baby less than 6 weeks old. Describe the main physical and behavioral features of the infant as you progress through the assessment. Are the features you describe appropriate for the infant's age?

5. Describe sleep wake states in which an infant is most receptive to latching onto the breast.

6. Practice using the New Ballard Score to determine the gestational age of a newborn baby.

7. Compare a neonate's mouth size, symmetry of shape, and tongue placement when she is at rest, is crying, and is well latched onto the breast. Describe normal characteristics of each.

8. A child's behavior while feeding at the breast changes as the child grows and develops. Act out how a 15-month-old child behaves while he is breastfeeding compared with a 2-week-old child.

9. Name at least one breastfeeding risk factor associated with an infant who is small for gestational age.

10. A preterm baby is one who is born before how many weeks? Does 1 or 2 weeks of prematurity affect a baby's breastfeeding abilities? If so, what is the effect? What assistance should the lactation consultant be prepared to offer?

C H A P T E R

21

FERTILITY, SEXUALITY, AND CONTRACEPTION DURING LACTATION

Fertility, sexuality, contraception, and lactation mutually interact in both physiological and psychological ways. A lactation consultant must understand these interactions before she can respond to inquiries about sexual relations and contraception during the breastfeeding interval. Questions in this chapter will help you to assess your understanding of this body of information and how it applies to professional practice.

Chapter Outline

Fertility

    The demographic impact of breastfeeding

    Mechanisms of action

    Lactational amenorrhea

    The suckling stimulus

    The repetitive nature of the recovery of fertility

    The Bellagio Consensus

Sexuality

    Libido

    Sexual behavior during lactation

Contraception

    The contraceptive methods

Clinical Implications

Summary

Key Concepts

References

Multiple-Choice Questions

1. When a mother breastfeeds at least seven times daily, ovulation is reliably prevented.

    a. True only in exclusively breastfeeding well-nourished mothers.

    b. False even in exclusively breastfeeding well-nourished mothers.

    c. True in all mothers in the second 6 months of the child's life.

    d. False except in exclusively breastfeeding under-nourished mothers.

2. The link between supplementing a breastfed infant and return of menses in the infant's mother is that

    a. the daily amount of suckling falls below some threshold amount needed to suppress ovulation.

    b. the imminent return of menses is accompanied by a marked decrease in breastmilk volume that prompts use of supplements.

    c. breastmilk loses much of its nutritive value after menses return.

    d. the infants who are most apt to receive supplements are older than 6 months, when menses are going to return shortly anyway.

3. The Bellagio Consensus contends that exclusive breastfeeding, in the absence of vaginal bleeding after the 56th day postpartum, provides

    a. about 75 percent protection against pregnancy during the second 6 months postpartum.

    b. about 75 percent protection against pregnancy during the first 6 months postpartum.

    c. at least 98 percent protection against pregnancy during the first 6 months postpartum.

    d. about 15 percent protection against pregnancy during the second 6 months postpartum.

4. Which of the following delays first ovulation and subsequent risk of pregnancy in a breastfeeding mother?

    a. infrequent infant suckling

    b. intense infant suckling

    c. supplementation of the infant's diet with other milks

    d. liberal use of pacifiers

5. When one assesses postpartum return of fertility, vaginal bleeding in the breastfeeding woman in the early weeks following birth

    a. indicates that her menses have returned.

    b. can usually be ignored unless it is very heavy.

    c. indicates that ovulation has occurred.

    d. indicates she has resumed sexual intercourse too soon.

6. Luteinizing hormone

    a. is secreted by the posterior pituitary.

    b. concentrations are low in lactating postpartum women and help to suppress ovulation.

    c. concentrations are high in lactating postpartum women and help to suppress ovulation.

    d. release is promoted by intense infant suckling.

7. Lactational amenorrhea alone will lower the rate of a subsequent pregnancy in a lactating woman to
   a. less than 3 percent.
   b. about 3 to 10 percent.
   c. about 12 to 15 percent.
   d. about 20 to 25 percent.

8. Liquid supplements offered to a breastfeeding infant are unlikely to promote ovulation in the mother until the supplements make up more than _____ percent of total feeds.
   a. 5   c. 15
   b. 10   d. 25

9. The duration of a breastfeeding mother's current lactational amenorrhea is
   a. directly related to the number of times a thriving baby breastfeeds in 24 hours.
   b. directly related to the duration of a previous period of lactational amenorrhea.
   c. inversely related, in a general way, to household income.
   d. inversely related to the mother's iron status.

10. Once menses resume after an interval of lactational infertility,
   a. the mother has ovulated or will do so the next month.
   b. the baby's diet must be supplemented because the mother's milk volume has dwindled.
   c. the mother can count on three or four more menstrual periods before ovulation.
   d. the baby's weight can be expected to plateau for about 3 weeks.

11. Low progesterone concentrations in the blood may be associated with feelings of
   a. relaxation.
   b. increased energy.
   c. "all's right with the world."
   d. vulnerability.

12. As compared with the amount of estrogen produced by bottle-feeding new mothers, a lactating woman usually produces
   a. lower concentrations.
   b. higher concentrations.
   c. about the same concentrations.
   d. concentrations that initially are about the same but then rise during the first 6 months.

13. The consensus among studies of the effect of breastfeeding on a sexual relationship strongly show that breastfeeding
   a. enhances the sexual relationship.
   b. detracts from the sexual relationship.
   c. has no effect on the sexual relationship.
   d. has no consistently predictable effect on the sexual relationship.

14. Hormonal contraceptives that contain estrogen cause breastmilk volumes to

    a. increase.

    b. decrease.

    c. neither increase nor decrease.

    d. increase in the early postpartum but decrease after about 4 months.

15. In women who wish to begin using hormonal contraceptives in the first 4 weeks postpartum, estrogen-containing contraceptives should be

    a. encouraged because they are effective.

    b. discouraged because they decrease maternal milk volume.

    c. encouraged because they promote a good letdown.

    d. discouraged because they increase the risk of maternal thrombosis.

16. With respect to the establishment of breastfeeding in the early postpartum, any delivery-room procedure, such as tubal ligation, that involves general anesthesia may

    a. delay breastfeeding because the anesthesia may be transferred in breastmilk and cause tonic bite in the baby.

    b. promote breastfeeding because of the extra nursing-staff attention that the mother will receive.

    c. delay breastfeeding because the mother is uncomfortable and may be separated from her infant.

    d. promote breastfeeding because it relaxes the mother.

17. The lactational amenorrhea method of contraception can be relied upon for contraception during the

    a. first 6 months postpartum.

    b. first 9 months postpartum.

    c. interval in which the baby is taking at least two breastfeeds per day.

    d. entire course of any breastfeeding.

18. Nonhormonal intrauterine devices used by lactating women

    a. are not more likely to be expelled because the woman is breastfeeding.

    b. reduce the leukocyte content of breastmilk.

    c. increase the likelihood of uterine perforation.

    d. decrease the time to first menses.

19. The use of estrogen-containing contraceptives by breastfeeding women is

    a. encouraged, because they are effective, and no steroid hormones are transferred into breastmilk.

    b. encouraged, because only insignificant amounts of hormones are absorbed by the infant.

    c. discouraged, because long-term effects of steroid consumption are unknown.

    d. discouraged, because the infant's metabolism multiplies the effect of ingested hormones.

20. Counseling for family planning is ideally provided

    a. before delivery with postpartum follow-up timed to match the method chosen.

    b. immediately after delivery, with follow-up within the first 2 weeks postpartum.

    c. after hospital discharge, with follow-up at the 6-week visit.

    d. after 6 weeks postpartum, following verification that breastfeeding is going well.

21. The earliest time to begin using progestin-only contraceptives while minimizing the risk of adversely affecting milk volumes is

    a. within 72 hours of delivery.

    b. after lactogenesis II is established.

    c. as soon as the milk has matured.

    d. 6 weeks postpartum.

22. The physiological trigger for the initiation of abundant milk production is

    a. withdrawal of progesterone.

    b. secretion of prolactin.

    c. withdrawal of estrogen.

    d. secretion of luteinizing hormone.

23. Types of contraceptives for lactating women, in order from most preferred to least preferred, are

    a. estrogen containing, progestin only, nonhormonal.

    b. estrogen containing, nonhormonal, progestin only.

    c. nonhormonal, progestin only, estrogen containing.

    d. nonhormonal, estrogen containing, progestin only.

24. In populations that do not use contraceptive technology, child spacing is determined principally by

    a. the mother's nutritional status, particularly protein adequacy.

    b. the incidence of illness in the family.

    c. the duration that each child is breastfed.

    d. the total number of children the couple plan to have.

25. As compared with bottle-feeding women, breastfeeding women in the early postpartum (less than 3 months)

    a. tend to have less pain during sexual intercourse.

    b. tend to delay resumption of sexual intercourse.

    c. commonly have more interest in sexual intercourse.

    d. prefer sexual intercourse more frequently.

26. Barrier contraceptive devices such as a diaphragm or cervical cap should not be fitted until some time after

    a. 3 weeks postpartum.

    b. 6 weeks postpartum.

    c. 3 months postpartum.

    d. when exclusive breastfeeding ends.

Discussion Questions

1. What are the relationships among contraception, fertility, sexuality, and lactation?

2. What are examples of a hormonal contraceptive? of a permanent nonhormonal contraceptive? of a nonpermanent, nonhormonal contraceptive? What is the effect of each type of contraceptive on breastfeeding?

3. For women in a developing region, what are the advantages and disadvantages of each type of contraceptive described in question 2? Are the advantages and disadvantages the same for women living in industrialized regions?

4. What criteria must be met for the lactational amenorrhea method of contraception to function optimally?

5. What is the effect of infant suckling on continued milk production? on the inhibition of ovulation? Is total minutes of suckling per 24 hours the only consideration, or does spacing throughout the 24 hours have an effect too?

6. When menses return, is the lactation amenorrhea method of contraception still sufficient? Why or why not?

7. What roles do gonadotropin-releasing hormone and luteinizing hormone play during the normal menstrual cycle of a nonlactating woman? Are concentrations of these hormones different in a lactating woman?

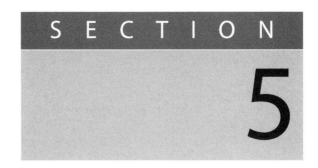

SOCIOCULTURAL AND RESEARCH ISSUES

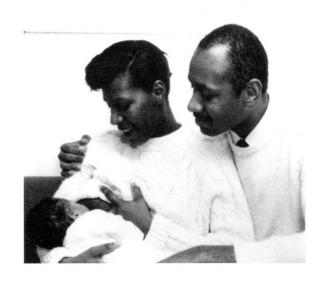

22

Research, Theory, and Lactation

If we are to make the best possible recommendations about breastfeeding management, we must have the best possible information about the physical, emotional, and social milieus of breastfeeding. How is that information obtained and analyzed? Lactation consultants must understand how to interpret findings reported in the published literature on breastfeeding and how to decide if the conclusions are clinically relevant. Questions in this chapter will help you to assess your understanding of this body of information and how it applies to professional practice.

Chapter Outline

Multiple-Choice Questions

1. Evolutionary theory is a framework for research that proposes that human biological phenomena
   a. are fixed; their purpose or bodily benefit do not change with time.
   b. change rapidly (usually within a few generations) to meet changing human needs.
   c. may have developed to serve needs in the distant past that are less obvious today.
   d. are highly variable in their response to changing environmental conditions.

2. One goal of qualitative research is
   a. gathering data that test a previously developed theory.
   b. investigating a broadly defined topic in greater detail.
   c. determining independent variables.
   d. detailed descriptions of people's experiences.

3. Grounded theory refers to a method

   a. used to understand beliefs, practices, and behavior patterns within the context of a particular culture or subculture.

   b. that describes behaviors influencing a person's perceived ability to complete a task.

   c. that explains actions as a function of the intention to perform the action.

   d. that generates theories based on people's interpretations of their own experiences.

4. Correlational studies examine

   a. relationships among the variables studied.

   b. only variables that vary directly with each other.

   c. only variables that vary inversely with each other.

   d. qualitative data.

5. One requirement of an experimental study is that

   a. data are collected at the nominal (naming) level.

   b. no intervention is used.

   c. at least one independent and one dependent variable is used.

   d. study subjects may come from a convenience sample.

6. While planning a medical research study, an investigator must

   a. avoid reading previous literature on the topic, so that others' conclusions will not be an influence.

   b. wait to state a hypothesis until after some of the data have been collected.

   c. determine the research method to use.

   d. determine how to obtain subjects without revealing the goal of the research.

7. The factor believed to control changes in an outcome variable is called a(n)

   a. quasi-dependent variable.

   b. intervention variable.

   c. independent variable.

   d. superior variable.

8. Factors for which the investigators did not control, but which exert an influence on the outcome variable, are called

   a. shadow variables.

   b. confounding variables.

   c. recruited variables.

   d. grounded variables.

9. When a null hypothesis is written, it is phrased to say that

   a. a significant negative relationship exists between the dependent and independent variables.

   b. a significant negative relationship does not exist between the dependent and independent variables.

    c. no variable other than the planned independent variable is likely to affect the outcome variable.

    d. the action of the independent variable will make no difference in the treatment group as compared with a control group.

10. Operational definitions explicitly describe

    a. how equipment used in the study is to be used and maintained.

    b. how the major variables in the study are defined.

    c. the purpose for which instruments such as questionnaires were devised.

    d. the basic parameters of the study, such as number of subjects to be recruited and length of time that subjects will be followed.

11. The MOST important reason that studies of the relationship between breastfeeding and infant health arrive at different conclusions is that

    a. the number of infants tracked may differ.

    b. the length of time that infants are tracked may differ.

    c. mothers of tracked infants may be reluctant to participate at follow-up.

    d. "breastfeeding" may be defined in different ways.

12. A person participating in medical research must

    a. be told something about the study.

    b. receive a full explanation of the particular treatment he or she will receive.

    c. agree to participate for the duration of the entire study.

    d. agree to allow responses to be tied to personal identifiers.

13. An investigator can fulfill her obligation to obtain informed consent from a study candidate by fully describing the study

    a. orally and receiving an oral consent.

    b. in writing and receiving an oral consent.

    c. orally and receiving a written consent.

    d. in writing and receiving a written consent.

14. Probability sampling is used when

    a. investigators recruit subjects for a qualitative study.

    b. investigators in a pilot study recruit subjects most likely to demonstrate the hypothesis being tested.

    c. few subjects are available and it is probable that nearly all must be recruited.

    d. subjects are chosen at random from the entire population of possible subjects.

15. Statistical analysis of the results of an experimental study that uses too small a sample size may

    a. not detect differences that actually exist between treatment groups.

    b. not detect apparent similarities that actually exist between treatment groups.

    c. reject the null hypothesis if an inverse relationship exists between independent and outcome variables.

    d. reject the null hypothesis if a positive relationship exists between independent and outcome variables.

16. The "reliability" of a study's results refers to the

    a. trustworthiness of the investigators.

    b. appropriateness of statistical methods used.

    c. accuracy and repeatability of measurements or observations over time.

    d. accuracy and stability of equipment used to make instrumental measurements.

17. "Validity" of a study's results refers to the degree to which

    a. the collected data are in fact true.

    b. the information generated by the study is clinically useful.

    c. the null hypothesis is rejected.

    d. the hypothesis tested is substantiated.

18. Findings in a study that the investigator did not anticipate

    a. mean that the study was not properly designed at the outset.

    b. can be the basis for other research in the future.

    c. usually result only when the investigator scans the data for a relationship not specifically tested for.

    d. should not be published.

19. In a published report, discussion of the limitations of a study

    a. undermines the study's credibility and should be avoided.

    b. should describe previously published reports on the topic.

    c. evaluates the degree to which the study's results can be generalized.

    d. should emphasize the strengths of the study's design.

20. The type of investigation generally recognized as providing the most sound basis for clinical practice is

    a. qualitative research.

    b. retrospective chart reviews.

    c. the case series.

    d. randomized, prospective trials.

Discussion Questions

1. What are the differences between qualitative and quantitative research? What kind of data are produced by each type of research? What is a research question that can be investigated by each type of research?

2. What are the main differences between descriptive, correlational, and experimental research methods? What is a research question that can be investigated by each type of research?

3. What research methodology is considered the most rigorous and the most likely to give valid results?

4. What is the difference between a sample and a population? Are investigators more apt to collect information from samples or populations?

5. What are the rights of human subjects in a research study? How are those rights protected? What if the subjects are breastfeeding infants?

6. What is the difference between an independent variable, a dependent variable, and a confounding variable? How does an investigator minimize the effect of confounding variables?

7. What is an "operational" definition? Does it differ from an ordinary dictionary definition? If so, why?

8. How can a review of literature help an investigator decide whether to pursue qualititative or quantitative research?

9. What is the difference between probability sampling and nonprobability sampling as ways to obtain subjects for a study? What is an example of each sampling method?

10. What is meant by reliability and by validity? To what aspect of research does each apply?

11. What is meant by interrater reliability, intrarater reliability, test-retest reliability, and internal consistency? What is an example of each?

12. According to one investigator, breastfeeding duration was longest when the mother had previously breastfed, had a full-term baby, and was married; however, parity trended in the opposite direction. Match each factor in the left-hand column with the appropriate descriptor in the right-hand column:

   1. marital status   a. dependent/outcome variable

   2. parity   b. independent variable

   3. previous breastfeeding experience   c. confounding variable

   4. breastfeeding duration

   5. full-term infant

13. As methods of collecting data, what are the strengths and weaknesses of interviews, field observations, and document review? In what kind of study is each method appropriately used?

14. Is a valid conclusion drawn from a well-designed research study necessarily clinically useful? How do you decide?

BREASTFEEDING EDUCATION

Whether talking to one person or to an entire roomful, lactation consultants teach. It is the heart of their job. Doing so effectively requires an understanding of the characteristics of adult learners. Questions in this chapter will help you to assess your understanding of this body of information and how it applies to professional practice.

Chapter Outline

Educational Programs

    Distance learning and Web courses

Learning Principles

Adult Education

Curriculum Development

Parent Education

Prenatal Education

Early Breastfeeding Education

    Continuing support for breastfeeding families

How Effective is Breastfeeding Education?

Teaching Strategies

Small Group Dynamics

Multimedia Presentations

    Slides

    Transparencies

    Television, videotapes, DVDs

    Compact disks

Educational Materials

    Education for at-risk populations

    Adolescents

    Older parents

Educational Needs and Early Discharge

Continuing Education

    Objectives and outcomes

The Team Approach

    Childbirth educators

    Nurses

    Lactation consultants

    Physicians

    Dietitians

    Community support groups

Summary

Key Concepts

Internet Resources

References

Multiple-Choice Questions

1. A new mother who attends prenatal breastfeeding classes and receives attention from a lactation consultant in the early postpartum is more likely than another mother to

    a. delay the baby's first feeding.

    b. feel overwhelmed with information.

    c. extend the period before weaning.

    d. feel ambivalent about breastfeeding.

2. A teachable moment refers to a moment when a learner

    a. debates a point with the instructor.

    b. experiences an "A-ha!" moment during which new information is understood and assimilated.

    c. feels a need for new information or skills.

    d. is confronted by a situation in which she must instruct other learners.

3. An adult tends to learn most efficiently when

    a. he works on his own at exercises that permit focused attention.

    b. students are not directly involved in the topic, so they have some perspective on it.

    c. information is sequenced in the order most useful to the instructor.

    d. the class requires active participation of students.

4. Kinesthetic learning occurs when the learner

   a. hears material, as when attending a lecture.

   b. touches or handles equipment or models.

   c. reads new information.

   d. uses as many senses as possible to incorporate new knowledge.

5. Adults in a class differ from children in which of the following ways?

   a. Adults are thinking primarily of others.

   b. Time is considered an abundant asset.

   c. The theoretical underpinnings of an action must be clearly explained.

   d. Education must be applicable to real life.

6. The MOST important principle, of those listed below, of adult education is to

   a. present information in large, comprehensive blocs.

   b. provide specific feedback at a later date, to reinforce student learning.

   c. provide take-home handouts instead of individualized assessment.

   d. mesh the information presented with students' readiness to learn that information.

7. As compared with their own prepregnant state, in the very early postpartum mothers retain new cognitive information

   a. better because the baby's presence sharpens perceptions.

   b. worse because of the physical and emotional intensity of childbirth.

   c. better because their pregnancy hormonal state has resolved.

   d. worse because of a hormonal mechanism related to "fight or flight."

8. Attendance at breastfeeding education programs by the baby's father or grandparents should be

   a. encouraged because they can attend to the new baby while the mother focuses on the instruction.

   b. discouraged because of the extra side conversations that result.

   c. encouraged because they influence the mother's ability to breastfeed.

   d. discouraged because they commonly express incorrect notions about breastfeeding.

9. In order to teach information that health-care providers think a new breastfeeding mother should know, the provider must first

   a. demonstrate her own expertise.

   b. address the mother's immediate concerns.

   c. demonstrate her own authority.

   d. address issues that the provider thinks are important.

10. For optimal learning and change in behavior, the ideal group size ranges from

    a. 1 to 5 persons.

    b. 4 to 8 persons.

    c. 8 to 12 persons.

    d. 10 to 15 persons.

11. Retention of a newly taught skill or bit of information is increased by

    a. hearing it only, so learners can focus on the instructor.

    b. seeing it only, so learners can focus on the instructor.

    c. practicing it only, so learners can focus on their own motor responses.

    d. using all sensory methods to learn.

12. Good information to discuss in a prenatal breastfeeding class is

    a. how to differentiate between pathological and physiological jaundice.

    b. the benefits of putting the infant to breast within an hour after birth.

    c. treatment of breast abscess.

    d. how to clip a newborn's fingernails.

13. Which of the following items is MOST important to teach breastfeeding mothers before postpartum hospital discharge? How to

    a. determine infant's gestational age.

    b. estimate infant's nutritional status.

    c. obtain assistance if the mother has questions.

    d. avoid diaper rash in the infant.

14. Booklets describing how to breastfeed that emphasize difficulties, discomfort, and inconvenience are more likely to

    a. prepare the mother for the realities she will face.

    b. be prepared by companies that sell manufactured baby milks.

    c. be prepared by organizations that promote breastfeeding.

    d. be prepared by organizations that support breastfeeding mothers.

15. Well-written breastfeeding education booklets

    a. are written at the reading level of the specific audience who will receive them.

    b. depict mothers of the social groups most likely to breastfeed.

    c. emphasize basic anatomy and physiology of lactation.

    d. are well balanced and thus describe and depict bottle-feeding also.

16. The attention and advice of peer counselors–lay women trained to help other breastfeeding women in their own communities–have been shown to

    a. have no particular effect on breastfeeding rates.

    b. increase breastfeeding initiation but not duration.

    c. increase breastfeeding initiation and duration.

    d. have no effect on initiation but to increase duration.

17. A behavioral objective typical of a continuing education program in breastfeeding management is as follows:

    a. The learner will state three early signs of infant hunger.

    b. The learner will understand the relationship between water supplements and incidence of jaundice.

    c. The learner will be able to recognize three signs of infant dehydration.

    d. The learner will learn how to elicit the proper infant gape for good infant attachment to the breast.

18. Mother-to-mother breastfeeding support groups are intended to provide

    a. a template for assuring long-term breastfeeding.

    b. a structured roadmap for managing early feedings.

    c. social and practical support for the breastfeeding mother.

    d. comparative descriptions of local physicians' attitudes toward breastfeeding.

Discussion Questions

1. How do adult learners differ from school-age learners? How should methods to teach about breastfeeding be modified to meet the needs of adult learners?

2. What is a teachable moment?

3. What is the difference between visual, auditory, and kinesthetic learning modes? Pick a single breastfeeding education topic and show how each mode might be used in teaching that topic.

4. What are at least three criteria that apply to printed educational materials that promote breastfeeding?

5. How might people in each of the following positions contribute to a program to educate hospital staff on optimal management of breastfeeding?

    a. perinatal nurses

    b. childbirth educators

    c. dietitians

    d. lactation consultants

    e. volunteer breastfeeding support group leaders

    f. physicians

6. What are modifiable maternal characteristics or situations that predict breastfeeding outcome? Which variables can be influenced by education of the mother? by education of labor and delivery room staff? How would you accomplish that?

7. Collect samples of breastfeeding education brochures designed for mothers. Evaluate the following aspects of each brochure:

    a. reading level

    b. compliance with WHO Code recommendations

    c. support of breastfeeding (general and specific)

    d. positive promotion of breastfeeding

    e. negative comments about breastfeeding

    f. discussion of risks of feeding formula

    g. photographs or illustrations at variance with statements in the text

8. Will you use any of the brochures evaluated in question 7? Why or why not?

THE CULTURAL CONTEXT OF BREASTFEEDING

The pull may be centrifugal or centripetal, but the norms of the culture in which we grow up remain the axis around which we rotate. Lactation consultants must understand and respect other mothers' cultural norms with respect to breastfeeding. Questions in this chapter will help you to assess your understanding of this body of information and how it applies to professional practice.

Chapter Outline

The Dominant Culture

Ethnocentrism versus Relativism

Assessing Cultural Practices

Language Barriers

The Effects of Culture on Breastfeeding

    Rituals and meaning

    Colostrum

    Sexual relations

    Wet-nursing

    Other practices

    Contraception

    Infant care

Maternal Foods

    "Hot" and "cold" foods

    Herbs and galactogogues

Multiple-Choice Questions

1. A "culture"
   a. is a coherent set of values, beliefs, norms, and practices of a particular group.
   b. is learned only by classroom instruction.
   c. does not guide decisions and actions in any predictable way.
   d. implies knowledge limited to a small, select subgroup of a population.

2. Cultural attitudes exert how much influence on breastfeeding?
   a. little, because breastfeeding is a natural biological process
   b. little, because the baby just born into a given culture controls much of the success of breastfeeding
   c. a lot, because the cultural context strongly determines how and when the mother feeds her infant
   d. a lot, but only in cultures that rely on tradition rather than on research-based evidence

3. A galactagogue refers to any
   a. person who openly advocates breastfeeding.
   b. food believed to increase milk secretion.
   c. food believed to dry up a mother's milk.
   d. food that promotes the breakdown of galactose.

4. Deliberate weaning is practiced
   a. in nearly all cultures around the world.
   b. only in highly technological societies.
   c. only in the developing world when the mother becomes pregnant again.
   d. only in those cultures where breastfeeding is considered appropriate only for a few months.

5. The hot-cold theory of foods identifies foods as "hot" when they are
   a. heated just prior to being eaten.
   b. warm colors such as pink, orange, or red.
   c. considered more easily digested than "cold" foods.
   d. very highly spiced.

6. Cultural relativism refers to

   a. a belief that one's own culture embodies the only right way in which to live.

   b. an appreciation of one's relatives and how they live and work.

   c. recognizing that all cultures share the same values.

   d. an appreciation and acceptance of different cultural norms.

7. When a lactation consultant evaluates breastfeeding practices of a client from a different culture, which question does she NOT need to ask?

   a. Is it helpful?

   b. Is it common?

   c. Is it harmful?

   d. Is it harmless?

8. Effective rituals

   a. reflect a belief in the efficacy of a particular ceremony.

   b. have been rigorously analyzed and shown to have the desired result.

   c. require adherence to traditional forms.

   d. are beyond the ability of Western science to explain.

9. Which of the following is sensitive to cultural norms?

   a. signs of dehydration

   b. time at which milk comes in

   c. age at which the infant is able to metabolize cereals

   d. age of the infant when table foods are added to his diet

10. A woman who immigrates to the United States from Southeast Asia and who has some children born abroad and some in the US is likely to

    a. breastfeed all of her children.

    b. bottle-feed all of her children.

    c. breastfeed children born abroad but bottle-feed children born in the US.

    d. bottle-feed children born abroad but breastfeed children born in the US.

11. To avoid being thought the cause of *mal de ojo* in an Hispanic infant, a lactation consultant should

    a. not look the infant in the eyes.

    b. not touch the infant's fontanel.

    c. look at the mother immediately after gazing at the child.

    d. touch the infant while she admires him.

12. In most cultures, meat

    a. plays a major role in the diet of a pregnant woman.

    b. plays a major role in the diet of a lactating woman.

    c. usually means beef.

    d. plays a minor role in the diet of the lactating woman.

Discussion Questions

1. What is the definition of *culture?*

2. What is the difference between allopathic and folk medicine? What is an example of a belief that typifies each?

3. As you evaluate unfamiliar breastfeeding practices, how might you categorize them in order to focus on which practices to support and which to attempt to modify?

4. What is an example of a common practice that is potentially harmful to a breastfeeding baby? How might you attempt to modify that practice?

5. What might be the underlying physiological reasons for a 40-day period of seclusion after childbirth?

6. What are complementary proteins? How do they figure into the diet?

7. What are some food restrictions or preferences practiced by women in various cultures during the post-partum period? What purposes are served by these restrictions or preferences?

8. What is meant by foods that are described as "hot" or "cold"? What cultures categorize foods in this way? How are foods in these categories used to maintain health?

9. What is the difference between gradual, deliberate, and abrupt weaning? What circumstances might prompt each type of weaning?

10. What developmental milestones are used in various cultures to indicate an appropriate time for weaning a child?

11. How is colostrum viewed in various cultures? Is it always the first feed of a newborn? Why or why not?

FAMILIES

It is not just mothers and babies who breastfeed; the entire family breastfeeds in the sense that family members must in various ways accommodate the breastfeeding dyad. For too many women, however, the family may be incomplete or a source of danger. Questions in this chapter will help you to assess your understanding of this body of information and how it applies to professional practice.

Chapter Outline

Multiple-Choice Questions

1. When a second child joins a household consisting of a mother, father, and older sibling, how many relationships now exist between these four individuals?

   a. 3   c. 6

   b. 4   d. 10

2. When is a discussion of infant feeding most effective in influencing a woman's decision to breastfeed?

   a. after the baby's birth

   b. after the mother has returned home

   c. during the prenatal period

   d. after the father starts showing an interest in breastfeeding

3. Significant others in a breastfeeding mother's life who support her breastfeeding usually

   a. are necessary for long-term breastfeeding.

   b. are nice but not necessary to continued breastfeeding.

   c. are best kept at a distance, because they just get in the mother's way.

   d. try to undermine the close breastfeeding relationship.

4. Of the following items, a first-time breastfeeding mother MOST needs which in order to continue breastfeeding?

   a. a helper to straighten up the house

   b. supplementary income

   c. a health-care provider knowledgeable about optimal breastfeeding practices

   d. friends who themselves are breastfeeding

5. Lactation consultant advice and teaching can influence a client's

   a. intention to breastfeed.

   b. socioeconomic status.

   c. attitudes toward her birth family.

   d. previous breastfeeding experience.

6. Lactation consultant advice and teaching can influence a client's

   a. age.

   b. previous infant-feeding experiences.

   c. social support.

   d. degree of formal education.

7. When a father has a new baby, he usually first touches the neonate with

   a. his fingertips, as he strokes the baby's arm or leg.

   b. his entire hand, as he holds the baby up.

   c. his fingertips, as he strokes the baby's chest.

   d. his face, when he offers a welcoming kiss.

8. One study suggests that the frequency of a father's visits to a hospitalized premature infant is

    a. about the same as the frequency of the mother's visits.

    b. directly correlated with infant weight gain.

    c. inversely correlated with paternal involvement with the infant several months later.

    d. unrelated to later infant development.

9. In general, adolescent mothers follow the same breastfeeding pattern as adult women in that

    a. their breastfeeding initiation rates are about the same.

    b. older teen mothers are more likely to breastfeed than younger teen mothers.

    c. their breastfeeding continuation rates are about the same.

    d. each subsequent child is breastfed for fewer months.

10. The likelihood of a low-income woman breastfeeding is increased if

    a. the baby's father supports breastfeeding.

    b. she lacks a high-school diploma.

    c. her maternal grandmother bottle-fed.

    d. she begins prenatal care in the third trimester.

11. A lactation consultant who believes that a client is being physically abused by someone with whom she lives has an obligation to

    a. sympathize but limit her actions to breastfeeding advice.

    b. overlook that evidence and try to make breastfeeding the bright part of the mother's life.

    c. counsel the mother about how to increase her safety and that of her infant.

    d. report her observations to child-protection authorities.

12. As compared with households in which infants are bottle-fed, households in which infants are breast-fed are likely to experience

    a. more household violence against women but not against children.

    b. less household violence against either women or children.

    c. more household violence against children but not against women.

    d. less household violence against women but not against children.

13. Of the following items, the strongest predictor that a mother will initiate and continue breastfeeding is

    a. high socioeconomic status.

    b. marriage to a man who supports breastfeeding.

    c. education beyond high school.

    d. the mother's intention to breastfeed.

Discussion Questions

1. What can a father do to grow close to his infant, other than feeding?

2. How does each of the following factors influence the likelihood that a low-income mother will breastfeed? that a high-income mother will breastfeed?

   a. racial or ethnic group

   b. degree of support

   c. access to information about lactation and breastfeeding

   d. hospital practices during labor and delivery in the postpartum

   e. use of manufactured baby milks by hospital staff

3. What factors are more likely to deter teenage mothers, as compared with older mothers, from breastfeeding?

4. Among low-income women, how do peer counselors influence breastfeeding initiation? duration of exclusive breastfeeding? total duration of breastfeeding? What makes the counselors successful?

5. Is there a relationship between breastfeeding and maternal feelings of empowerment? If so, what is the relationship, and what causes it?

ANSWER KEY TO MULTIPLE-CHOICE QUESTIONS

Chapter 1
1. a
2. b
3. c
4. d
5. b
6. d
7. b
8. b
9. c
10. a
11. a
12. c
13. b

Chapter 2
1. c
2. d
3. a
4. b
5. d

Chapter 3
1. b
2. b
3. c
4. d
5. a
6. a
7. d
8. c
9. b
10. d
11. b
12. b
13. a

14. d
15. a
16. a
17. d
18. c
19. a
20. b
21. a
22. b
23. a
24. b
25. d
26. d
27. a
28. c
29. b
30. b
31. b
32. a
33. c
34. d
35. a
36. b

Chapter 4
1. d
2. c
3. b
4. c
5. a
6. d
7. d
8. b
9. c
10. d
11. d

12. b
13. b
14. b
15. a
16. d
17. b
18. b
19. c
20. c
21. d
22. d
23. b
24. d
25. a
26. b
27. d
28. b
29. c
30. c
31. d
32. d
33. c
34. d
35. c
36. b
37. a
38. b
39. c
40. c
41. b
42. b
43. d

Chapter 5
1. b
2. d

3. b
4. c
5. d
6. b
7. b
8. c
9. c
10. d
11. d
12. d
13. b
14. c
15. a
16. c
17. a
18. d
19. b
20. a
21. a
22. c

Chapter 6
1. b
2. d
3. c
4. c
5. c
6. d
7. b
8. b
9. a
10. b
11. d
12. a
13. c

Chapter 7
1. a
2. a
3. b
4. b
5. a
6. d
7. b
8. c
9. d
10. b
11. d
12. b
13. c
14. c
15. c
16. c
17. b
18. c
19. b
20. b
21. b
22. d
23. d
24. b
25. d
26. d
27. c
28. a
29. d
30. a
31. d

Chapter 8
1. d
2. d

3. c
4. a
5. c
6. b
7. a
8. c
9. c
10. b
11. a
12. c
13. a
14. b
15. b
16. a
17. c
18. c
19. d
20. c
21. b
22. c
23. b
24. b
25. d
26. d
27. c
28. c
29. d
30. a
31. a
32. c
33. c
34. d
35. c
36. b
37. a
38. b
39. a
40. d
41. b

42. d
43. c
44. c
45. c
46. a

Chapter 9
1. b
2. a
3. c
4. d
5. b
6. d
7. c
8. d
9. c
10. d
11. d
12. b
13. d
14. c
15. a
16. b
17. d
18. c
19. b
20. b
21. d
22. c
23. b
24. c
25. a

Chapter 10
1. c
2. b
3. d
4. b
5. a
6. a
7. c

8. d
9. a
10. a
11. b
12. d
13. b
14. c
15. a
16. d
17. b
18. c
19. b
20. d
21. a
22. a
23. b
24. c
25. c

Chapter 11
1. d
2. a
3. b
4. a
5. a
6. d
7. a
8. d
9. c
10. a
11. c
12. a
13. a
14. d
15. c
16. c
17. b
18. b
19. c
20. a

Chapter 12
1. a
2. a
3. b
4. c
5. a
6. d
7. d
8. b
9. c
10. b
11. d
12. a
13. d
14. a
15. d
16. b
17. b
18. b
19. b
20. b
21. b
22. b
23. c
24. b
25. b
26. a

Chapter 13
1. a
2. c
3. b
4. b
5. a
6. c
7. c
8. a
9. b
10. c
11. c

12. d
13. a
14. d
15. b
16. c
17. c
18. d
19. b
20. b
21. d
22. c
23. c
24. d
25. d
26. c
27. b
28. d
29. a
30. c

Chapter 14
1. b
2. c
3. b
4. b
5. c
6. c
7. c
8. c
9. b
10. a
11. d
12. c
13. b
14. b
15. c
16. b
17. d
18. c
19. d

20. c
21. d
22. c
23. c
24. c

Chapter 15

1. b
2. b
3. c
4. c
5. b
6. a
7. b
8. c
9. a
10. d
11. d
12. d
13. c
14. d
15. c
16. d
17. b
18. c
19. c
20. c
21. d
22. c
23. d

Chapter 16

1. a
2. b
3. d
4. a
5. d
6. a
7. c
8. a
9. b

10. c
11. c
12. b
13. d
14. c
15. a
16. b
17. c
18. a
19. c
20. a
21. a
22. c
23. c
24. b
25. c
26. c
27. b
28. d
29. b
30. c
31. b
32. c

Chapter 17

1. c
2. b
3. b
4. a
5. c
6. c
7. d
8. b
9. a
10. b
11. a

Chapter 18

1. a
2. c

3. d
4. b
5. c
6. b
7. a
8. c
9. a
10. c
11. b
12. c
13. d
14. c
15. c
16. b
17. c
18. a
19. d
20. c
21. b
22. a
23. a
24. d
25. a
26. a
27. b
28. b
29. b

Chapter 19

1. d
2. b
3. d
4. b
5. a
6. d
7. a
8. d
9. d
10. a

11. a
12. d
13. a
14. b
15. c
16. a
17. d
18. b
19. d
20. c
21. b
22. c
23. b
24. d
25. c
26. b
27. a
28. c
29. a
30. b
31. d
32. b
33. c
34. b
35. d
36. b

Chapter 20

1. c
2. d
3. c
4. a
5. c
6. d
7. a
8. d
9. a
10. b
11. b

12. b
13. a
14. d
15. c
16. a
17. c
18. b
19. d
20. c
21. c
22. b
23. a

Chapter 21

1. b
2. a
3. c
4. b
5. b
6. b
7. b
8. c
9. b
10. a
11. d
12. a
13. d
14. b
15. d
16. c
17. a
18. a
19. c
20. a
21. b
22. a
23. c
24. c
25. b
26. b

Chapter 22

1. c
2. d
3. d
4. a
5. c
6. c
7. c
8. b
9. d
10. b
11. d
12. b
13. d
14. d
15. a
16. c
17. a
18. b
19. c
20. d

Chapter 23

1. c
2. c
3. d
4. b
5. d
6. d
7. b
8. c
9. b
10. c
11. d
12. b
13. b
14. b
15. a
16. c
17. a
18. c

Chapter 24

1. a
2. c
3. b
4. a
5. c
6. d
7. b
8. a
9. d
10. c
11. d
12. d

Chapter 25

1. c
2. c
3. a
4. d
5. a
6. c
7. a
8. b
9. b
10. a
11. d
12. b
13. d